WHAT NURSES KNOW...

MENOPAUSE

WHAT NURSES KNOW ...

MENOPAUSE

Karen Roush
RN, MS, FNP, BC

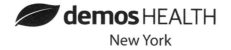
demosHEALTH
New York

Visit our web site at www.demosmedpub.com

Acquisitions Editor: Noreen Henson
Cover Design: Steve Pisano
Compositor: NewGen
Printer: Hamilton Printing

Medical information provided by Demos Health, in the absence of a visit with a healthcare professional, must be considered as an educational service only. This book is not designed to replace a physician's independent judgment about the appropriateness or risks of a procedure or therapy for a given patient. Our purpose is to provide you with information that will help you make your own healthcare decisions.

The information and opinions provided here are believed to be accurate and sound, based on the best judgment available to the authors, editors, and publisher, but readers who fail to consult appropriate health authorities assume the risk of any injuries. The publisher is not responsible for errors or omissions. The editors and publisher welcome any reader to report to the publisher any discrepancies or inaccuracies noticed.

Library of Congress Cataloging-in-Publication Data

Roush, Karen.
    What nurses know—menopause / Karen Roush.
       p. cm.–   (What nurses know)
    title: Menopause
  Includes bibliographical references and index.
    ISBN 978-1-932603-86-6 (alk. paper)
1.   Menopause–Popular works.   I. Title.   II. Title: Menopause.
RG186.R68 2011
618.1'75–dc22   2010028371

Special discounts on bulk quantities of Demos Health books are available to corporations, professional associations, pharmaceutical companies, health care organizations, and other qualifying groups. For details, please contact:

Special Sales Department
Demos Medical Publishing
11 W. 42nd Street
New York, NY 10036
Phone: 800-532-8663 or 212-683-0072
Fax: 212-941-7842
E-mail: rsantana@demosmedpub.com

Made in the United States of America
10 11 12 13   5 4 3 2 1

About the Author

Karen Roush, RN, MS, FNP, BC, has been a nurse specializing in women's health issues for over 25 years. She is a former Editorial Director of the American Journal of Nursing and is currently a Mary Clark Rockefeller Scholar and PhD candidate in the College of Nursing at New York University. She is also the author of the first book in this series, *What Nurses Know ... PCOS.*

WHAT NURSES KNOW...

Nurses hold a critical role in modern health care that goes beyond their day-to-day duties. They share more information with patients than any other provider group, and are alongside patients twenty-four hours a day, seven days a week, offering understanding of complex health issues, holistic approaches to ailments, and advice for the patient that extends to the family. Nurses themselves are a powerful tool in the healing process.

What Nurses Know gives down-to-earth information, addresses consumers as equal partners in their care, and explains clearly what readers need to know and want to know to understand their condition and move forward with their lives.

What Nurses Know titles are organized simply, with call-out boxes for "What Nurses Know..." special tips, fun facts, and things that only a nurse would know. Personal stories are interspersed throughout, so the reader can easily relate to the books.

Titles published in the series

What Nurses Know ... PCOS
Karen Roush

What Nurses Know ... Menopause
Karen Roush

Forthcoming books in the series

What Nurses Know ... Diabetes
Rita Girouard Mertig

What Nurses Know ... Multiple Sclerosis
Carol Saunders

What Nurses Know ... Chronic Fatigue Syndrome
Lorraine Steefel

Contents

Foreword

Nurses make great educators. They have a gift for truly understanding their patients' questions, concerns, and fears. Nurses are also typically in charge of making sure information about health conditions and medication instructions are clear. If you want an explanation that will make sense and be easy to understand—ask a nurse. Nurse Karen Roush skillfully tackles the often-confusing time in women's lives known as menopause in *What Nurses Know...Menopause*. Roush cuts through the hype to provide down-to-earth, medically proven information about this important transition time in a woman's life.

In *What Nurses Know...Menopause*, the reader learns

- She's not alone when she describes a variety of troublesome symptoms during menopause
- What menopause symptoms mean and how to effectively treat them

- How to keep yourself healthy throughout menopause—what screening tests are important and how to adjust lifestyle habits to changing needs during menopause
- Where to go for more information, including reliable Internet resources

Roush provides a detailed discussion about hormonal therapy and practical tips on when to consider hormone therapy, why hormone replacement can be beneficial, and how hormones are best taken. She also focuses on symptoms that truly add to the distress of menopause that may be glossed over during busy appointments with the gynecologist—like sleep disturbance, sexual dysfunction, and bone health changes. Roush describes how the woman's body changes during menopause and what's needed to keep in top shape during this period of transition.

Using her nursing background, Roush provides clear, practical instructions for using medications for a wide range of menopause symptoms. She likewise provides details on using supplements, alternative, and complementary nondrug treatments. *What Nurses Know...Menopause* is a one-stop shop for what most women want to know about menopause—what is it, why is it happening, what changes should I expect, how can I best control symptoms, and how do I keep myself healthy. The practical tips scattered through this book answer typical questions just when you begin to ask yourself, "But I wonder how I'm supposed to ...." Open this book, and you'll feel like you have your own personal nurse, walking you through this time of change.

Dawn A. Marcus, MD
Professor
University of Pittsburgh

Introduction

Menopause—frankly, I wasn't prepared for this. Even though as a Nurse Practitioner I helped countless women through the process, counseling and prescribing, and assuring them they would get through it. All the while thinking I would breeze through, I mean, really, isn't a lot of it mind over matter anyway? I'm fit and active and strong-willed, facing my passing years without too much angst. No hot flashes were going to intrude on my world.

And then it started. Slowly at first: a slight warm flush as I blow-dried my hair, one less cover on the bed at night. In fact, I welcomed these; they arrived in the middle of another long cold Adirondack winter. I remember opening up the bathroom window to let in the icy air, saying "All right, bring it on!" Then it stopped for awhile, and then came back a little stronger. Not so welcome this time, but still tolerable.

Then it changed. My menstrual cycle stopped and the anxiety attacks started. I have never had anxiety in my life, and at first

I didn't recognize what was happening. The sense of impending doom, the shortness of breath, the panicked feeling. Thoughts raced through my head: Something is terribly wrong, I'm having a heart attack, something horrible is going to happen, I'm going to die. I didn't notice at first that every attack preceded a hot flash. The anxiety would rise up, threaten to overwhelm me, then start to subside; and as it did the hot flash would start. Every single time.

And that is how it has continued. I have never had a hot flash without first having an anxiety attack and I have never had an anxiety attack that wasn't followed by a hot flash. Yet every single time the anxiety is so intense I think, "This time I am going to die, this time it's not a hot flash." During the worst of it I was having up to 40 of them a day. It was exhausting and debilitating. It sapped my energy, distracted me from my work. Every so often they would do a disappearing act, sometimes for a few months; and just when I was thinking I could celebrate, bam, they were back. Stress made it worse, fatigue made it worse, hot weather made it worse.

It's been five years and it has gotten better. Days go by without any attacks and unless I'm going through a particularly stressful time, rarely do I have more than two a day. Like the women I assured in my Nurse Practitioner practice, I'm getting through it.

During the height of perimenopause I went searching for a book that would help guide me through the process, not as a health professional but as a woman dealing with a difficult transition. But the nurse in me still needed to know that the information I got was up-to-date and based on the latest research. I couldn't find one that was straightforward and gave me the information I needed to make decisions. So that is why the second book of this series on *What Nurses Know...* is about menopause. I wrote the book I needed to help me through the last five years.

So read on. And hang in there. You too will get through it.

WHAT NURSES KNOW . . .
MENOPAUSE

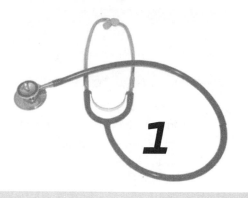

Menopause: An Overview

I expected menopause to be a joyous transition—and much later in life! How sadly disappointed I have been.   JOYCE

Menopause is not so bad. I thought I would be crazy or sad, but I feel pretty good.   CAROL

I think if you have trouble with getting older you might have more trouble with menopause, but it's part of your life; it's a journey. Sometimes I'd like time to slow down, but otherwise...   SUSAN

When my mother went through menopause, she had a lot of heavy, heavy bleeding; she couldn't even go out. Her doctor told her it was because of her hormones, so I was expecting the same thing. Instead, not a thing. I had my normal periods and then one day it stopped and I never had one again. And not getting my period anymore was a gift—I was so happy, I didn't care about anything else.   LIZ

Menopause has been described in many ways: the change of life, the climacteric, an ending, a beginning, the "death of woman-hood," freedom. It has been cursed and celebrated, dreaded and accepted. For some women it is a nonevent, for others it disrupts their lives. In our youth-obsessed society it can herald invisibility and becoming obsolete. Yet, in an era of increasing life expectancy it can also mean half a lifetime of new adventures and sexual freedom.

Menopause is a chronological event, reminding us that we are growing older. It is a physiological event, a herald of all kinds of age-related changes in our bodies. It is psychological, an indication of shifts in our roles as intimate partners and as mothers.

It is impossible to separate menopause from the context of our changing lives and increasing age. Think about what is happening as a woman approaches 50. We begin to face the reality of our own mortality. Visible signs of aging increasingly stare back at us from the mirror. Children leave home for college and homes of their own. We may find our careers shifting as a new crop of young careerists gain a foothold in the workplace. Retirement planning starts to take on an urgent significance. Intimate relationships shift or perhaps even end.

Yet this stage of life also holds potential benefits and exciting possibilities. Many women report increasing freedom to do what *they* want after putting children, partners, and parents first for so many years. They have greater self-confidence and a sense of accomplishment. And increased security about who they are, what they believe, and what they are doing gives them the freedom to speak up and go after what they want.

Many myths and misunderstandings have grown around menopause. If something happens between the age of 45 and 60, it gets blamed on menopause. Failed relationships, stalled careers, another dress size outgrown—blame it on menopause. Lack of estrogen is the ultimate scapegoat for every age-related problem women encounter, from wrinkles to Alzheimer's.

What is the truth about menopause? There is no one truth. Every woman experiences menopause differently. There are physiological changes all women will go through, dives and dips in hormones, and shrinking reproductive organs. But how you experience these will depend on the idiosyncrasies of your particular body, your life experiences, and your current life situation. It will be affected by when you were born; women who grew up as part of the baby boomer generation lived a different life than those born before World War II. Women's roles and expectations changed dramatically with the women's movement in the 60s and 70s. Different opportunities create different paths through life. Where you are in your 40s and 50s is partly a result of the social fabric that prevailed during different phases of your life.

But there are real choices to be made as you go through the menopausal transition. And there are new opportunities presenting themselves in this next phase of your life. Armed with accurate up-to-date information, you can be your own best guide through this "change of life." Change may feel uncomfortable at times, but it always offers new possibilities.

What We're Talking About When We Talk About Menopause: Defining Terms

"She's going through menopause."
"I can remember when my mother went through menopause."
"I've been going through menopause for four years now."

We often hear the term menopause used in this kind of context, as a process, something one *goes through*. We've probably said it ourselves many times. However, menopause is not actually a *process*. It is one point in time—the time of your final menstrual period (FMP). Menopause is defined as the permanent end of menstruation.

The word *menopause* comes from the Greek words *meno* (month) and *pausis* (cessation), which were first used to describe the end of menstruation.

The *process* that you go through as you approach the FMP is the *menopausal transition.* This encompasses the time from when your periods first start to change through that final period. This time period is also called *perimenopause* or less commonly, the *climacteric.*

Part of the confusion may come from the fact that 12 months have to go by without a period before the last period is determined to have been *the final* period. So you reach menopause 12 months before it can be determined that you did. In other words, you are postmenopausal for 12 months before you know for sure that you reached menopause.

• •

STRAW—Recommended Definitions

Following are the definitions of terms recommended by STRAW—the Stages of Reproductive Aging Workshop. STRAW was a workshop in July 2001 sponsored by the American Society of Reproductive Medicine, the National Institute on Aging, the National Institute on Child Health and Human Development, and the North American Menopause Society. The purpose was to develop a staging system for female reproductive aging and recommend standard language to describe the years around the time of menopause. The following definitions are taken from their Executive Summary.

Menopause—the point in time that is defined as 12 months of amenorrhea (no periods) following the FMP, which reflects a near complete but natural diminution of ovarian function.

Menopausal transition—begins with variation in menstrual cycle length in a woman who has a rise in follicle stimulating hormone and ends with the FMP (not able to be recognized until after 12 months of amenorrhea).

Perimenopause—literally means "about or around menopause." Encompasses same time period as menopausal transition. Should not be used in scientific papers, but only with patients and in the lay press.

Climacteric—popular but vague term that is synonymous with perimenopause and also should not be used in scientific papers, but only with patients and in the lay press.

Postmenopause—Divided into two stages: Stage +1 (early) and Stage +2 (late). The early postmenopause is defined as five years since the FMP, during which there is a further dampening of ovarian hormone function to a permanent level, as well as the period of accelerated bone loss. Stage +2 is from five years after the FMP until the woman's death.

We may also talk about *going through menopause* because many women continue to experience symptoms like hot flashes for years after their final period. So it certainly feels like you are *going through* something! Women equate postmenopause with the time after it has all stopped—periods, hot flashes, night sweats—and they are comfortable in the new phase of their lives.

The term *premenopause* can also be confusing and, in fact, NAMS and the Stages of Reproductive Aging Workshop (STRAW) both recommend discarding the term completely. Premenopause literally means *before menopause*, which would be the period of a woman's reproductive life from puberty to perimenopause. It is far too broad a time period to have meaning and, besides, to refer to an adolescent girl or 20-year-old woman as premenopausal is silly.

What is the meaning of menopause in the life of a woman? The answer to this question has changed over time as women's roles have changed and our life span has increased.

Menopause: From Nervous Disorder to Natural Part of Life to Disease of Deficiency

In 1900 the average life expectancy in the United States was 48 years for white women and 34 years for black women, so most women didn't live long enough to experience menopause, or if they did they were postmenopausal for only a short period of their lives. Today the average life expectancy for women is 81 years, so many of us will live 30 or 40 years after menopause, a third to half of our lives. It is not surprising that how women, the health care profession, and society in general view menopause has changed over the years.

A BRIEF HISTORY OF MENOPAUSE

The earliest mention of menopause goes way back to ancient Greece. The writings of Aristotle and others during this era note that reproductive ability ends in women with the cessation of menses, usually around 40 years of age and never beyond the age of 50. During the Middle Ages in Europe, from the 6th to the 15th century, there were numerous references in scholarly texts to the cessation of menses. Most put the permanent cessation of menses no later than the age of 50.

The first use of the term menopause was by a French physician, Charles de Gardanne, in 1816. At the time it was seen as a nervous disorder manifested in various physical and mental illnesses. In an 1845 book on female diseases, menopause was described as a time when a woman "ceased to exist for the species" and "resembled a dethroned queen." The first complete book on menopause, *The Change of Life in Health and Disease* by Edward Tilt, published in Britain in 1857, listed 135 different symptoms brought on by menopause. These included melancholia, hystericism, hysterical flatulence, "an abundant eruption of boils," pseudonarcotism, "uncontrollable peevishness," and temporary deafness. It was this book that coined the phrase, "change of life." It warned that all but a few women would suffer some form of mental health dysfunction during this time, which if neglected could lead to insanity.

In the United States in the early 1900s, menopause was generally not seen as a problem. Women's role was that of mother and then grandmother, and menopause was seen as an important milestone in a woman's life, not a distressing one. Estrogen was available in the form of ovarian extracts but it was in short supply and expensive. The medical consensus at the time seemed to be that menopause was a natural process and healthy living and education was all most women needed to make the transition smoothly.

Estrogen became more widely available in the 1940s with the production of diethylstilbestrol (DES), a synthetic hormone, and the development of a method for extracting estrogen from the urine of pregnant mares. However, menopause was still viewed by most experts as a natural milestone for women. In fact, there was more of a tendency to ignore women's suffering during perimenopause and after. The 1940s and 1950s was a time of rigid gender roles. Complaints of symptoms at menopause were usually seen as the melodramatic reactions of weak and irrational women. Husbands were often portrayed as victims, sent into younger women's arms by their menopausal wives' irrational behaviors. Attempts by women to enrich their lives were seen as desperate attempts to deny the reality of their situation, one of decline and loss.

None of this was supported by statistics; there was no uptick in the number of women experiencing psychiatric problems during menopause. Studies conducted during the 40s and 50s consistently found that the majority of women reported no major problems related to menopause. When women were asked what they considered the worst part of menopause, the most frequent answer had nothing to do with loss or physical symptoms. Most answered it was not knowing what to expect.

In the 1960s the publication of two best-selling books set the tone that would prevail throughout the next decade: *Everything You've Always Wanted to Know About Sex (But Were Afraid To Ask)* by Dr. David Reuben, a California psychologist, and *Feminine Forever* by Dr. Robert Wilson, a New York City gynecologist. *Everything You've Always Wanted to Know About Sex (But Were Afraid To Ask)* sold millions of copies. Millions of women read that, "having outlived their ovaries, they [had] outlived their usefulness as human beings." Forget about holding on to your sexuality because "as estrogen is shut off, a woman comes as close as she can to being a man." Reuben claimed that menopausal women "live in a world of intersex," not really a man or a woman.

Feminine Forever had an even greater impact on women's lives. It was this book and articles by Wilson published in medical journals that defined menopause as a deficiency disease that could and *should* be treated by estrogen treatment. (See Chapter 7 for more about *Feminine Forever* and estrogen.) Menopause put a woman in a state of "living decay" and her husband and family, in fact all of society, suffered as a result of her instability.

Women responded in different ways to these views of menopause. This was a time of shifting perspectives on women's roles. Feminism and the advent of the "pill" had far-reaching consequences for women of all ages. Being a wife and mother was no longer seen as central to a women's life. At the same time, when the focus shifted away from motherhood as the defining measure of a woman's value; youth, beauty and sexuality stepped into its place, bringing their own set of pressures for women.

Some women welcomed the attention given to menopause in the 60s and 70s, glad that at last a women's health issue was getting some serious interest. Others rejected the views as an attempt by the medical community to medicalize a natural life process. While some feminists viewed estrogen as a way for women to have control over their bodies, others saw it as attempts by the medical community and drug companies to make money off of women's health. These different views were also reflected in the popular literature of that time. Magazine articles ranged from those that encouraged women to think of estrogen the same way they think of hair dye to cover their gray, to those that told women there was no reason to use estrogen for the "natural" process of menopause.

From the 60s to early 70s the experience of menopause and use of estrogen therapy (ET) continued to be tightly woven together. In the mid-70s, studies linked estrogen to endometrial cancer and estrogen briefly fell out of favor. Then it was discovered that adding progestin took care of that risk, and once again menopause became something a woman could avoid with the use of estrogen-plus-progestin therapy.

In her 1991 book, *The Silent Passage*, Gail Sheehy spoke of menopause as "the last taboo" in a time when everything else was open to discussion. That changed throughout the 90s as the baby boomers entered their 40s and 50s. They redefined aging and menopause along with it. Women who had come of age in the 60s were not about to allow themselves to be relegated to a graceless old age. The information age saw the change from patient to health care consumer and women made the most of it. They armed themselves with information and became active decision makers when it came to menopause. Estrogen became one option among many—natural products, exercise, yoga, and dietary measures—to manage menopause. Women read about menopause, talked about menopause, and even laughed about menopause. In 2001, 10 years after *The Silent Passage* was first published, a highly successful musical comedy opened in Orlando, Florida, *Menopause The Musical*. It went on to hundreds of performances all over the world and continues to be performed to sell-out crowds to this day. Menopause is not a taboo subject any longer!

Getting Informed

There is a tremendous amount of information about menopause out there today. There are women's organizations, support groups, books, magazine articles, and Web sites. And don't forget your health care provider. Talk to him or her and keep talking throughout the menopausal transition and onward. This is an ongoing active process and a health care provider you trust is a valuable guide through it.

What Nurses Know...

Not all information is good information. There is a lot of information on the Internet that is inaccurate, outdated, or biased. Pay attention to the organization the information is coming from. Is it an educational institution, government agency, nonprofit organization, or for-profit business? If products are recommended, take a second look to see if the Web site was developed by the company producing the products. Is the Web site really just a vehicle to promote a product, book, or service? What are the credentials of the person writing the information? When was the information last updated? This book features a list of resources at the end of each chapter that includes trustworthy Web sites.

At the end of each chapter you will find a list of reliable Internet resources. There is new information coming out all the time, so keep checking back periodically to stay informed with the most up-to-date information.

Resources

MayoClinic.com

Clinicians at the Mayo Clinic provide information on many topics through this Web site, including menopause.
www.mayoclinic.com/health/menopause/DS00119

MedlinePlus

This government Web site is a service of the National Institutes of Health. It has links to a large number of informational sources. Information is available in 12 languages.
www.nlm.nih.gov/medlineplus/menopause.html

North American Menopause Society (NAMS)

NAMS is a nonprofit professional organization dedicated to promoting menopause-related health and quality of life. It does this through research, education, and resources for women and health care providers. Their Web site has comprehensive information on menopause for women, as well as a menopause clinician search tool. Information is available in English, Spanish, and French.
www.menopause.org/

Pause

This Web site by The American College of Obstetricians and Gynecologists (ACOG) offers comprehensive information in a consumer-friendly format. It also has a physician locator tool.
http://pause.acog.org/

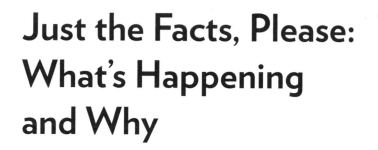

Just the Facts, Please: What's Happening and Why

The Menopause Transition

So, what is actually happening during this menopausal transition? And what is behind all the changes your body is undergoing? To understand the changes that happen with the reproductive system during the menopausal transition you must first understand what's been happening all the years before menopause. First, a quick review of the reproductive system and the menstrual cycle.

The Female Reproductive System

The reproductive system consists of internal organs, external genitalia, and various hormones. Breast tissue may also be considered part of the reproductive system because it is involved in the hormonal changes associated with menstruation and reproduction, and because of its role after childbirth. Following is a quick review of the reproductive organs.

The internal reproductive organs sit inside the pelvis and include the vagina, uterus, ovaries, and fallopian tubes.

The *vagina* (Latin for "sheath" or "scabbard") is a muscular tract that extends from the cervix (narrow lower part of the uterus) to the external genitalia. It is not an open hollow tube; its sides remain collapsed in on themselves until something is inserted into it, like the penis during sexual intercourse. During our reproductive lives, the vagina is three to four inches long and the vaginal walls are elastic and moist.

The *uterus* (Latin for "womb") is a hollow, pear-shaped muscular organ about the size of your closed fist. It is lined with the endometrium, which thickens and then sloughs off during each menstrual cycle.

The *ovaries* are two oval-shaped glands, one on each side of the uterus, each measuring about one-and-a-half inches long. They store and release eggs. The ovaries also secrete hormones and are the body's main source of estrogen. (Small amounts of estrogen are also produced by peripheral fat cells.)

The *fallopian tubes* are two narrow tubes that extend about four to six inches from the uterus to the ovaries. They are not attached to the ovaries but open into the abdominal cavity very close to them. Hair-like projections called cilia "catch" the egg when it is released from the ovary and move it down the tube to the uterus. Conception happens in the fallopian tube.

The *external genitalia* consist of the labia majora, labia minora, and the clitoris. The labia majora ("large lips") are the fleshy outer skin flaps. They envelope and protect the other external genitalia. The labia minora ("small lips") are the smooth smaller inner skin flaps surrounding the vaginal opening. The clitoris is a small, sensitive erectile organ at the upper meeting point of the labia minora. The clitoris has 8,000 nerve endings and is the site of the female orgasm. The term *vulva* encompasses all of the external genitalia.

Hormones are chemical substances in your body that are produced and secreted by specific glands or organs and then move via the blood to act on another part of the body. They act as messengers or triggers but do not have any activity of their own; their function is to regulate the activity of their target cells. The hormones primarily involved in the reproductive system are gonadotropin-releasing hormone (GnRH), follicle stimulating hormone (FSH), luteinizing hormone (LH), estrogen, progesterone, and testosterone.

The secretion of reproductive system hormones works in what is called a negative feedback loop. In a negative feedback loop, when levels of a hormone get too high they trigger a message to the appropriate gland to slow down or stop secretion. When the level falls below a certain amount, another message goes out and secretion picks back up again.

The menstrual cycle is controlled by the secretion and withdrawal of hormones. It has two phases: the follicular (proliferative) phase and the luteal (secretory) phase. The whole process begins in the hypothalamus gland in the brain. It produces GnRH, which in turn stimulates the pituitary gland to secrete the gonadotropins, FSH, and LH. FSH and LH then direct the ovaries to secrete estrogen and progesterone.

ESTROGEN

There are three types of estrogen produced naturally by our bodies: estradiol, estrone, and estriol. Estradiol is the major form of estrogen during our reproductive years. It is made primarily by cells in the ovaries. Estrone and estriol are produced in fat cells and the adrenal glands. Estriol is the weakest of the three and is produced in large amounts by the placenta during pregnancy. Outside of pregnancy it is present only in small amounts that don't change with menopause. After menopause, the adrenal glands and fat cells are the primary sources of estrogen, and estrone is the major type of estrogen produced.

Estrogen attaches to receptors on cells of its target tissues. The primary target tissues are those of the uterus and breasts. It also acts on bone, brain, blood vessel, kidney, liver, and intestinal tissues.

Estrogen causes a number of different actions in target tissues. It stimulates the growth of some tissues, such as the endometrium in the uterus, and milk ducts and connective tissue in the breasts. It increases collagen production. Collagen is connective tissue; it forms the matrix that supports and strengthens skin, bone, muscles, and other tissues. Estrogen limits the action of osteoclasts, cells that break down bone. It indirectly influences control of the liver's production of high-density lipoproteins (HDLs, the "good cholesterol") and low-density lipoproteins (LDLs, the "bad cholesterol").

Estrogen also acts on tissues in ways that can have a negative effect. It increases the potential for blood clotting. Its stimulation of uterine and breast tissue can increase the risk of uterine and breast cancer. These actions underlie some of the risks associated with hormone therapy.

TESTOSTERONE

There is another hormone involved in the reproductive system—testosterone. Testosterone is the major androgen. Androgens are hormones commonly referred to as the male sex hormones; they are responsible for male characteristics and reproductive activity. Males make and use high levels of them. However, women produce androgens as well, just in lesser amounts and for different purposes. (And yes, males produce small amounts of estrogen as well.) Androgens play a big role in a girl's transition to puberty, and throughout a woman's life they are important in estrogen production, bone health, and sexual desire.

In females, androgens are produced by the ovaries and the adrenal gland, with the ovaries responsible for 50 percent of the testosterone produced. Testosterone levels fall gradually as you get older so that by age 45 you have about half the level of testosterone you did when you were in your twenties. Levels continue to fall after menopause but not dramatically. It is thought that the falling level is related to age rather than menopausal status.

The ovaries continue to produce some testosterone throughout the postmenopausal years.

The Menstrual Cycle During The Reproductive Years

PHASE 1: FOLLICULAR

The menstrual cycle begins on the first day of a woman's period. Estrogen and progesterone levels are at their lowest, cuing the hypothalamus to secrete more GnRH, which signals the pituitary gland to secrete FSH and LH. This causes several follicles in the ovaries to begin to mature. Each follicle contains an egg. The developing follicles produce inhibin B, a protein which signals back to the pituitary gland to hold FSH production. As FSH levels decrease, only a single follicle continues to mature. The mature follicle produces estrogen, which peaks on about the twelfth day of the cycle. Stimulated by increasing amounts of estrogen, the lining of the uterus thickens and develops a richer blood supply. When the level of estrogen peaks there is a surge in LH, which then triggers the release of an egg (ovulation) within one to two days.

PHASE 2: LUTEAL

The cycle now enters the luteal or premenstrual phase, generally from day 14 to day 1 of the next period. Under the influence of LH, the follicle develops into a temporary body known as the corpus luteum (yellow body). The corpus luteum secretes estrogen and increasing levels of progesterone, which increases the thickening of the endometrium. This prepares the uterus to accept an embryo when conception occurs. If fertilization does not occur, the corpus luteum shrinks, estrogen and progesterone production decreases, and the drop in progesterone causes the lining of the uterus to slough off. The woman's period begins and the whole process starts over again.

During a woman's reproductive years, the average menstrual cycle takes 28 days, but a range from 25 to 35 days is considered normal. Bleeding lasts an average of five days with a normal range of three to seven days.

The Menstrual Cycle During The Menopausal Transition

The menopausal transition is a complex process, but if there is any one thing that *causes* menopause, it is the increasing loss of ovarian follicles over time. This loss actually begins at birth and continues at a varying rate throughout our lives. At birth, our ovaries contain 1 to 2 million follicles. By the time we reach menopause there are only about 1,000 follicles left in the ovaries. The number of follicles steadily decreases from birth until about age 37 when there is an increasingly rapid loss of follicles. Most are lost through a natural process called follicular atresia—the follicle breaks down and is reabsorbed by the body. Only about 500 follicles are lost through monthly ovulation over our lifetime.

As women enter perimenopause, the rate of follicular loss accelerates even more and the remaining follicles become less responsive to FSH stimulation. The pituitary responds by sending increased amounts of FSH and LH to try and stimulate egg production. The decreased number of developing follicles also means less inhibin B to hold off FSH production, which also contributes to increased FSH production. The increased number of follicles maturing is a factor in the rapid rate of follicle loss during this time. For awhile, the increased number of follicles maturing keeps the estrogen level up—remember that mature follicles secrete estrogen—sometimes even higher than what it was prior to perimenopause.

As the menopausal transition continues, fewer follicles mature, resulting in less estrogen being produced. Estrogen levels drop 6 to 12 months before menopause. After menopause, a small amount of estrogen continues to be produced in peripheral fat tissue.

Early transitional changes are unpredictable. Studies have shown that hormone levels during the menopausal transition vary significantly, not only among different women but also for each individual woman at different times in the menstrual cycle. At times, FSH may be at normal reproductive age levels and at other times it is elevated to levels you would expect to see in postmeno-pausal women. Ovarian function does not slow down in a smooth, gradual process. Follicles may not respond to FSH for months, then a follicle will start to mature. That is why during this transitional time your periods may be so irregular or you may go for months without any, only to have them return right on schedule for a few months. That is also why you can still get pregnant.

You may notice that as your periods become more irregular, the bleeding becomes heavier. This is because when ovulation does not occur there is continued estrogen production but no drop in progesterone to trigger the endometrium to shed, resulting in a thicker build-up. When you do ovulate and have a period, the shedding of this thicker lining is what causes the heavy bleeding.

Changes in the Reproductive Organs

The reproductive organs change in a number of ways during the menopausal transition. Along with other changes, they all get smaller in size. Some changes are related to the aging process, not menopausal changes. In fact, it is hard to separate out what changes are directly related to menopause from those that are directly related to the aging process.

VAGINA
The vagina shortens and loses elasticity (vaginal atrophy). Vaginal tissue thins and becomes drier. The vaginal fluid becomes less acidic, a factor in the increased susceptibility of older women to urinary tract infections (see Chapter 9 for more information on urinary health).

UTERUS
The uterus shrinks in size and becomes fibrotic (muscle tissue hardens). The cervix gets smaller as well, and in some women who are not sexually active the cervical opening will narrow or close completely (cervical stenosis).

OVARIES

The ovaries shrink and, as discussed earlier, the number of follicles decreases dramatically. By menopause the ovaries are about
half the size they were during peak reproductive years and can
no longer be felt by your health care provider when she or he does
the internal part of your gynecological examination.

EXTERNAL GENITALIA

Both pairs of labia lose underlying fat tissue and become smaller.
There is decreased blood flow to the entire area as well as atrophy of
the smooth muscle tissue of the clitoris, affecting its erectile function. (For a full discussion of sex and menopause see Chapter 5.)

BREAST TISSUE

Milk ducts in breast tissue no longer have estrogen to stimulate
them, so they atrophy as well, resulting in decreased breast size.
Breast tissue also becomes less dense with more fatty tissue. Loss of
connective tissue means less support for the breasts, so they sag.

Going Through the Menopausal Transition: Time and Duration

The menopausal transition usually lasts from five to ten years, more
often closer to five years. Subtle early signs of perimenopause actually begin when a woman is in her thirties but are first noticed by

What Nurses Know...

Stat Fact

*It is estimated that 6,000 women in the United States reach
menopause every day.*

women in their forties. The average age when women reach menopause (the time of the final menstrual period) is between 50 and
52 years, but can range from 45 to 55 years of age. Smokers are likely
to go through perimenopause two years earlier than nonsmokers
and are also likely to have a shorter menopausal transition.

Most women experience the menopausal transition as
described in the previous section. Their periods become more and
more irregular with changes in the duration and amount of bleeding. They may have regular periods for a while, followed by months
without one. Then, often once a women is convinced they're gone
for good, they're back. Nearly 10 percent of women abruptly stop
having a period. They may miss a period or two over a six- or nine-
month period, and then, nothing; they are gone. Or they may never
skip a period; one month they have a regular period and the next,
nothing. And that's it. They've hit menopause. (Though they won't
know for sure until twelve months later.)

Early or premature menopause is defined as natural menopause at age 40 or younger. This is menopause that happens

What Nurses Know . . .

*There is a "normal" range of experiences when it comes
to going through menopause. The norm is determined by
studying many women's experiences and finding the average
or most common experience. The average falls in the middle
of what is called the* normal distribution, *the well-known bell
curve. However, with any bell curve there are always "normal"
experiences on the extreme outer edges in both directions. If
you fall outside the "normal" or "average" experience, it does
NOT mean that you are abnormal or that there is necessarily
anything wrong with you.*

naturally, not as a result of surgery or other treatments, like chemotherapy. Premature menopause usually results in more severe symptoms and increased risk of osteoporosis and cardiovascular disease. The loss of fertility in premature menopause can be devastating to women who have waited to start or who have not yet completed their family.

Induced Menopause

Induced menopause refers to menopause that is brought on by something other than a natural decrease in ovarian function over time. The most frequent causes of induced menopause are surgical removal of the ovaries and chemotherapy or radiation treatments for cancer, most commonly breast cancer.

Chemotherapy will induce menopause in 53 to 89 percent of women being treated for breast cancer with commonly used chemotherapy regimens. Certain drug combinations will suppress

What Nurses Know...

Early or premature menopause is not the same thing as premature ovarian failure *or* hypothalamic amenorrhea.

Premature ovarian failure *is a decline in ovarian function that results in amenorrhea (no periods) in women younger than 40 years of age. Common causes are autoimmune diseases, genetic abnormalities, and chemotherapy. It is usually permanent.*

Hypothalamic amenorrhea *is a decline in ovarian function brought on by over-exercising, high levels of stress, or an eating disorder. This is a temporary condition; once the causes are resolved normal periods usually return.*

ovarian function, leading to estrogen depletion and induced menopause. Women being treated with similar chemotherapy drugs for other types of cancer, such as Hodgkin lymphoma, also experience induced menopause. The likelihood of chemotherapy-induced menopause increases after the age of 35 and approaches 100 percent after the age of 45. Ovarian function may return over time in some women, but for most, menopause is permanent.

Cancer treatment that includes radiation to the abdominal or pelvic area causes damage to the ovaries and can result in loss of ovarian function. The higher the radiation dose, the more likely you will experience induced menopause.

Surgical menopause happens after a woman has both ovaries removed in a surgical procedure. The medical term for this is *bilateral oophorectomy*. Most are done as part of a hysterectomy. Even when the ovaries are not removed, women who have a hysterectomy tend to experience menopause about five years earlier than women who don't have a hysterectomy.

When women have a hysterectomy they are often given the choice to have their ovaries removed at the same time. One of the reasons for removing the ovaries is to prevent the need for further surgery later on. A small percentage of women who have a hysterectomy have repeat surgery afterward to remove the ovaries, most often due to pelvic pain. The reported rates range from less than 1 percent to as much as 9 percent of women.

Another reason to remove the ovaries is to prevent ovarian cancer. Ovarian cancer is the fourth most common cause of cancer deaths. There is no way to screen for ovarian cancer and symptoms are so vague and nonspecific that it almost always goes undetected until too late. It is estimated that 1,000 new cases of ovarian cancer could be prevented if woman over 40 having a hysterectomy had their ovaries removed during the procedure. However, if you are not at an increased risk of ovarian cancer then you are probably better off keeping your ovaries. In 2007, a group of researchers reviewed studies that looked at mortalities of women with and without oophorectomies and found that in women who had hysterectomies between the ages of 50 and 54 there was an 8 percent decreased likelihood of living until age 80 if they had had their ovaries removed.

Early menopause has its risks. The ovaries are a major producer of androgens as well as estrogen. The ovaries continue to produce androgens after menopause. Androgens are involved in the production of estrogen in fat cells. When ovaries are removed you have a much sharper drop and greater reduction in both estrogen and testosterone levels. This often results in more severe symptoms like hot flashes, lack of sexual desire and response, and fatigue.

What Nurses Know...

Stat Facts

- *About 20 million women in the United States have had a hysterectomy*

- *About 600,000 women undergo a hysterectomy every year*

- *More than a quarter of women in the United States will have a hysterectomy by the time they are 60 years of age*

- *Hysterectomy is the second most frequent major surgical procedure that reproductive-aged women in the United States undergo (cesarean section is the first)*

- *The three most common reasons for a hysterectomy are fibroid tumors, endometriosis, and uterine prolapse*

- *More than half of women who have a hysterectomy before the average age of natural menopause have both their ovaries removed*

- *In women aged 45 to 55 years who had a hysterectomy, 76 percent had both ovaries removed*

In fact, women who have "induced menopause" from any cause experience more severe symptoms. Instead of estrogen production slowing down over time, it drops suddenly. Studies indicate that women who undergo induced menopause, whether from chemotherapy or surgery, have worse hot flashes and higher estrogen use than women who undergo natural menopause.

Resources

American Association of Clinical Endocrinologists (AACE)

AACE is an organization of physicians specializing in endocrinology. They offer a search tool—Physician Finder—that will list endocrinologists practicing in your area.

www.aace.com/org/ (Home page of AACE)

www.aace.com/resources/memsearch.php (Physician Finder)

Centers for Disease Control and Prevention (CDC)

Department of Health and Human Services

The CDC has a Web site on menopause. It has links to numerous resources on menopause topics.

www.cdc.gov/reproductivehealth/WomensRH/Menopause.htm

North American Menopause Society (NAMS)

NAMS is a nonprofit professional organization dedicated to promoting menopause-related health and quality of life. It does this through research, education, and resources for women and health care providers. Their Web site has comprehensive information on menopause for women, as well as a menopause clinician search tool. Information is available in English, Spanish, and French.

www.menopause.org/

Pause

This Web site by The American College of Obstetricians and Gynecologists (ACOG) offers comprehensive information in

a consumer-friendly format. It also has a physician search tool.
http://pause.acog.org/

womenshealth.gov
This government-sponsored Web site is part of the National Women's Health Information Center. It contains comprehensive information about menopause.
www.womenshealth.gov/

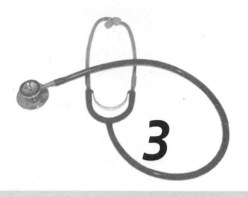

3

Hot Flashes and Night Sweats

I read that hot flashes are supposed to go away after your periods stop completely. Well, I've had hot flashes for five years now and haven't had a period for the last four of them. In fact, they got a lot worse after my last period. It's been only in the last few months that they've begun to subside.   KRISTINE

I had no idea it could be so debilitating. When they describe a hot flash as the feeling of being in a 450-degree oven, that's no exaggeration. It's like being hit in the solar plexus—the whole body is involved. You're flushing and sweating in places that make you so uncomfortable. You can't focus. It leaves you feeling completely ZAPPED.   HOPE

Of all the symptoms associated with menopause, hot flashes and night sweats (otherwise known as vasomotor symptoms) are probably the worst. They are certainly the one that women complain about the most, and with good reason. A full-blown hot flash leaves you flushed, sticky, distracted, and frustrated. If you have ever gotten out of the shower feeling fresh and clean in the morning only to find yourself feeling stale and sticky before you're even finished dressing, you know the feeling. Or stood on a bus or subway in the middle of a February cold spell, peeling off every piece of clothing you could without getting arrested for indecent exposure, you know the feeling. Or sat in a business meeting using your quarterly report as a fan hoping no one will notice the sweat dribbling down your face, you know the feeling.

Night sweats are hot flashes during the night, accompanied by perspiration. The experience of night sweats is highly variable for women; from not awakening at all, to waking with a damp pillow, to needing to change soaked sheets in the middle of the night. Regardless of severity, night sweats disrupt sleep and steal your energy. It is hard to be on top of your game when your sleep is interrupted night after night. Not to mention the effect it can have on your sex life and intimacy.

About 70 percent of women will experience hot flashes during menopause. They are usually most severe during the perimenopausal period and taper off after menopause. There are many women out there who will argue with that, though, because for some hot flashes and other symptoms will continue long after they throw away the half-empty box of sanitary pads in the back of the closet.

Some women are lucky enough to go through menopause without a single hot flash, or experience only mild occasional flashes. For others they are severe, sapping their energy and disrupting their life. Studies find that women with the most bothersome hot flashes are the ones most likely to suffer anxiety and depression during perimenopause and after menopause. Hot flashes are the reason most women used hormone therapy (HT) in the past and continues to be so today. (For a full discussion of HT, see Chapters 7 and 8.)

For most women, hot flashes start early in perimenopause and peak just before their last period. However, this is not the experience for everyone. A third of women have hot flashes for up to five years after menopause and for some they persist for as long as 15 years. A small number, about 20 percent, will still be having hot flashes into their 70s and 80s. Women who have surgical menopause are more likely to suffer severe hot flashes over a longer period of time.

Most hot flashes are brief, lasting about four minutes on average. (Though when a hot flash is severe, few women would describe four minutes as "brief.") They can last up to 10 minutes and in rare cases even longer. Though the experience is highly variable among women, it usually does not vary for the individual woman. Once a pattern is established it will probably stay consistent throughout the experience.

What Causes Hot Flashes?

The jury is still out on exactly what causes a hot flash. It is thought that the hypothalamus is the culprit. The hypothalamus regulates the body's temperature. During a hot flash it is thought that the hypothalamus reacts to a false sense that you are too warm and goes into action to cool you down. It dilates the blood vessels near the skin's surface to send more blood where it can dissipate body heat. It triggers perspiration so the body can cool itself off. It may also increase your

What Nurses Know...

Menopause is not the only thing that causes hot flashes. Some medications may cause hot flashes. Thyroid disease, infections, and certain cancers also can cause hot flashes. Talk to your health care provider about any unusual symptoms that accompany hot flashes, any change in the pattern of hot flashes (once established the pattern usually stays pretty consistent), or a new onset after an extended period of time without hot flashes.

heart rate, circulating the blood more rapidly to the surface to be cooled.

Certain medications can cause hot flashes. Among these are a group of drugs that many women may find themselves taking during this time of their life, selective estrogen receptor modifiers (SERMs). Tamoxifen is a SERM commonly used for the treatment of breast cancer and raloxifene (Evista) is prescribed for women with osteoporosis. If hot flashes become overwhelming while on these medications, talk to your health care provider about adjusting your dose or trying a different treatment.

Who Gets Hot Flashes?

There is no way to know who will and who won't experience hot flashes. There is no particular body type or personality that increases or decreases your chances of experiencing hot flashes. Some studies have suggested that women who are heavier are more likely to have hot flashes, whereas others suggest the opposite. It doesn't matter if your mother or sister had them or not. Sisters will often have very different experiences with the menopause transition.

Currently, there is nothing you can do to decrease the likelihood you will experience hot flashes when you transition to menopause. Staying fit, eating a healthy diet, and decreasing stress in your life are all important and valuable for many reasons; unfortunately, preventing hot flashes in menopause is not one of them.

There are some studies that suggest that postmenopausal women who have a longer history of hot flashes and are using HT may have more cardiovascular disease affecting the aorta (the largest artery in the body). The reason for this is not understood; it may have more to do with duration of HT than with the persistence of the hot flashes.

On the other hand, night sweats have been found to be associated with an almost 30 percent lower risk of death from any cause over the next 20 years, regardless of a woman's risk factors. There is still so much we don't understand about hot flashes; research continues on these and all aspects of vasomotor symptoms.

Strategies

There are numerous strategies that women use to control or cope with hot flashes, some with more success than others. There are lifestyle changes, medications, and alternative therapies. However, if you're looking for strategies backed by scientific evidence, there are few out there. Most are prescription medications, including HT;

What Nurses Know...

Off-Label Prescribing

The Food and Drug Administration (FDA) does not give blanket approval for any medication. It is approved for specific uses only. After approval the FDA works with the drug's manufacturer to agree on the drug's labeling—specific information about usage including indications, dosage, and administration. Labeling describes in detail the FDA-approved usage of the drug and is based on what clinical trials have shown to be safe and effective.

When a drug is prescribed for something other than an approved use, it is called off-label prescribing. Health care providers use their professional judgment, expertise, and experience when they decide to prescribe something off-label. This practice is common and legal. There is debate among health care professionals, pharmaceutical companies, and regulatory agencies about the practice.

Your provider should always let you know if they are prescribing a drug off-label and discuss it in-depth with you. If you think an off-label use of a drug may be beneficial to you, gather information about it to share with your health care provider and open a discussion with them about using it.

selective serotonin reuptake inhibitors (SSRIs), a class of drugs used for the treatment of depression; gabapentin (Neurontin), a drug used for epilepsy and migraines; and certain drugs used for the treatment of high blood pressure. Though there is some research to support the effectiveness of all of these, HT is currently the only one that is approved by the FDA for the treatment of hot flashes. However, the other medications are frequently prescribed off-label for the treatment of hot flashes.

Other than prescription medications, there is some evidence that black cohosh, a North American herb, may be effective, though more research is needed before conclusions can be made. The only other strategy with research that supports its use is acupuncture. Research results were mixed until recently, when studies have found more evidence that acupuncture is an effective treatment for many women.

Lifestyle Changes

Sometimes you can avoid hot flashes by avoiding certain triggers. Common triggers include heat, alcohol, hot drinks, spicy food, caffeine, and stress. If you're not sure what your triggers are, keep a record of your hot flashes for a month. Note what you were doing immediately before the hot flash started, any food or beverage you had just eaten, and your emotional state.

I found it really helpful to avoid the triggers; for me that's anxiety, wine and chocolate. HOPE

Being in a hot environment or in a stressful situation makes them worse. I love wine but I have more hot flashes when I drink, so I mostly avoid it. FRAN

Once you've identified your triggers the trick is to do something about them. Some things are easy to avoid, such as spicy food or a hot drink. Other things you may not have as much control over, such as the temperature outside or even inside, in your office space for example. And some things you have more control over than you may think, like stress.

In the middle of the winter I'd be wearing my sleeveless shirt under a button down sweater so I could take the sweater off. I'd be sleeveless in the middle of winter with the windows wide open! SUSAN

TIPS FOR STAYING COOL WHEN THE TEMPERATURE IS HOT

- Dress in layers
- Dress in lightweight cotton fabrics or self-wicking materials
- Carry a collapsible fan everywhere
- Get a mini fan for travel
- Keep a bottle of body spray in the fridge
- Keep pillow cases in a plastic bag in the freezer
- Partially freeze the water in your water bottle

TIPS FOR REDUCING STRESS

- Exercise regularly
- Do yoga or tai chi
- Meditate
- Develop a destressing routine, such as relaxing with music and candles or walking in the woods
- Keep a journal
- Take a good hard look at your schedule and consider rearranging where appropriate

Medications

HORMONE THERAPY

The truth is nothing works like estrogen to control hot flashes. There are many alternatives out there and some woman find significant relief with them, but none have been shown to be as effective as HT.

HT is FDA-approved only for *short-term* treatment of severe hot flashes (it is approved for long-term use only in the treatment of osteoporosis). Risks increase significantly the longer you are on it and the farther out from menopause you are.

Taking HT is a personal decision. Each woman has to weigh the risks and benefits for herself, in counsel with her health care provider. For a full discussion of the risks and benefits associated with HT, see Chapter 7, Hormone Therapy: What We Know Now and What It Means For You.

SELECTIVE SEROTONIN REUPTAKE INHIBITORS

Selective serotonin reuptake inhibitors (SSRIs) are medications that act on chemicals in the brain to relieve depression and anxiety. Research supports their use for the relief of hot flashes as well. This includes the drugs fluoxetine (Prozac), sertraline (Zoloft), paroxetine (Paxil), and citalopram (Celexa), among others. Some of the more common side effects of SSRI medications include drowsiness, dizziness, headache, sleep problems, vivid and strange dreams, apathy, changes in appetite, weight loss or gain, and sexual problems. Many people find if they can hold out a couple of weeks the side effects improve. This is only if the side effects are mild or moderate. You should not continue a medication with intolerable side effects.

It usually takes about four weeks for the medication to work. If you are not getting a good response by six weeks it is unlikely that you will. If you do decide to stop taking the medication, you must stop it gradually or you will get withdrawal symptoms. Though SSRIs are not addictive, they can cause symptoms like dizziness, headache, nausea, and diarrhea when they are stopped, especially if they are stopped all at once.

GABAPENTIN

Gabapentin (Neurontin) is a drug of many colors. It was initially approved by the FDA for treatment of seizure disorders and has since been used off-label for anxiety, muscle pain, migraine headaches, and schizophrenia. Now add hot flashes to the mix. There is evidence that gabapentin is effective for relief of hot flashes. In clinical trials women taking gabapentin reported greater relief of their hot flashes than women taking a placebo. Symptom relief happens in about four weeks.

If you haven't had relief much beyond that time, it is unlikely that you will.

The most frequent side effects of gabapentin are dizziness and somnolence (extreme sleepiness) or fatigue. About 10 to 15 percent of women stop taking the drug due to these side effects. If you can wait it out, they usually let up after a few weeks. Starting on a low dose and slowly increasing it can help as well. Other less common side effects include rashes, heart palpitations, and edema of the hands and feet. Once you stop the drug, all of the side effects go away.

Acupuncture

Acupuncture is a technique used in traditional Chinese medicine for thousands of years. Acupuncture uses needles to stimulate certain points on the body along pathways called meridians. The exact mechanism at work is not known. The National Institutes of Health and the World Health Organization recognize acupuncture as an effective component of health care management.

According to traditional Chinese medicine, hot flashes may be caused by deficiencies in the kidney or liver, or both, and a yin/yang imbalance. Needling sites may be determined on an individualized basis depending on where symptoms indicate the deficiency is, or it may be a standardized set of sites thought to affect hot flashes. The treatments usually last about 30 minutes. Most people find the treatment painless.

Studies of acupuncture and hot flashes have had mixed results. Some studies showed that acupuncture decreased hot flash frequency and severity, whereas others found no difference between women who received true acupuncture and women who received sham acupuncture. Sham acupuncture is a procedure where needling is done but the sites for needle insertion are believed to have no effect on hot flashes. Some studies have shown that women who received the sham acupuncture reported the same improvement in symptoms as women who received the true acupuncture. Whether this was a placebo effect or there is some benefit from simply the needling procedure is unknown. The latest research has been more positive, finding significant improvement of symptoms with the use of acupuncture.

Another positive research finding related to acupuncture treatment for hot flashes is that, unlike with HT, the effects do not vanish once you stop the treatment. Women continued to benefit for 6 to 12 months afterward.

Dietary Supplements

There are a number of dietary supplements that women use to treat hot flashes with varying success. Among the most common are phytoestrogens (plant estrogens), black cohosh, ginseng, dong quai, and evening primrose oil.

When using dietary supplements, keep in mind that there is little scientific evidence that they actually work. Either they have not been studied or, if they have been, the studies are too small or not conducted well enough to really give us accurate, dependable information. Studies not only tell us if something works, but also reveal possible harmful effects.

Another consideration is that dietary supplements are not approved or regulated by the FDA. This means that there is no control over what the labels say, what quality control measures are in place, or how dosage consistency is assured.

PHYTOESTROGENS

Phytoestrogens are estrogen-like compounds found in plant sources. They have a structure similar to estrogen and may be able to bind to estrogen receptors and produce weak estrogen effects. There are three main types: isoflavones, lignans, and coumestans.

Isoflavones   Isoflavones are a type of phytoestrogen found in legumes and beans. They appear to act similar to SERMs in their estrogen activity, that is, they promote estrogen activity in some tissues and suppress it in others. Soybeans are an excellent source of isoflavones. Other sources of isoflavones include:

- Lentils
- Kidney beans
- Lima beans
- Chickpeas

There is mixed evidence about the effectiveness of soy products in relieving hot flashes.

Part of the problem lies within the studies themselves; it is difficult to ensure that the type and dose of isoflavones are the same for study participants and across studies. Recent studies that looked at a specific dose of an extract of genistein, one of the primary isoflavones in soy foods, found it to be very safe and effective in managing hot flashes.

There are many options for adding soy to your diet. Along with soybeans and tofu there are now hundreds of soy products, including milk, cheese, burgers, and bars. You can also get genistein as an over-the-counter (OTC) supplement.

If you have a history of breast cancer or are at high risk for breast cancer, talk to your health care provider before increasing your dietary intake of isoflavones. There have been some concerns that soy foods can stimulate the growth of existing tumors. The most recent research suggests that this is not the case, but research is continuing; ask your health care provider for the latest information.

Lignans and Coumestans Lignans and coumestans are not as widely used for relief of menopausal symptoms because they do not have the same estrogenic effect or broad application as isoflavones.

Lignans come from whole grains and fruits and vegetables. Flaxseed is the best source of lignans. The best sources for coumestans are clover seeds and alfalfa sprouts.

BLACK COHOSH
Black cohosh is a North American herb. The World Health Organization does recognize it as a treatment for hot flashes and the North American Menopause Society recommends it for

What Nurses Know...

You've probably heard the term "placebo effect" many times. What does it actually mean in scientific terms? It refers to a well-documented phenomenon where people involved in a study who are in the control group, those not receiving the intervention but instead receive a drug or action that looks like the intervention, report the same desired effects as those receiving the actual intervention.

women with mild hot flashes. Study results have been mixed. A number found it to be beneficial in treating hot flashes, whereas some found little difference between women taking black cohosh and those taking a placebo. Many of the studies were conducted poorly, making their results unreliable.

There are concerns about a small number of reports of liver toxicity in menopausal women using black cohosh. Most studies show no serious bad effects with use. Better research is needed before a connection between black cohosh and liver disease can be confirmed or rejected. Until then you may want to ask your health care provider to do a blood test to check your liver function before you start taking black cohosh. The most common side effects women report after taking it are gastrointestinal (GI) upset and headaches. There is no information on the effects of long-term use and until this information is available you should use black cohosh for short-term use only.

Most studies of black cohosh have been done with a German product called Remifemin. Since this product has been studied more extensively than others, it is a good first choice.

GINSENG

Ginseng is an Asian root that has been used since ancient times for many purposes. There is very little research about

What Nurses Know ...

Treat supplements like you would any medication. Put them on the list of medications you are taking. Talk to your provider about them and go over possible interactions with medications you are already taking.

its use for hot flashes, and what there is has not shown any benefit. There are a few reports of postmenopausal bleeding in women who used it and it can interact with warfarin therapy (Coumadin).

DONG QUAI

Dong quai is a Chinese herb used to treat many disorders over many centuries. There is no evidence that it relieves hot flashes and it is not used in traditional Chinese medicine for that purpose. There is also no information on its safety, including any effect on the endometrium or risk of breast cancer. It can interact with warfarin (Coumadin).

EVENING PRIMROSE OIL

Evening primrose oil comes from the seeds of the evening primrose plant, a North American wildflower. Only one study looked at the use of evening primrose oil for relief of hot flashes and it found no benefits. There are no known safety concerns with its use, though some women complain of GI symptoms when taking it.

Behavioral Strategies

Some women have found relief using behavioral methods like paced respiration and relaxation techniques. Paced respiration is basically slow, deep breathing. Training can be done with biofeedback or on your own. Paced respiration uses diaphragmatic breathing, which means breathing using the muscles of your abdomen instead of the muscles of your chest. Inhale for three to five seconds, then exhale for three to five seconds, keeping your chest still. Do paced respiration for 15 minutes twice a day and when you feel a hot flash coming on. This has the added benefit of being great for relieving stress!

Resources

MayoClinic.com

Clinicians at the Mayo Clinic provide information on many topics through this Web site, including menopause. There is a section specifically on hot flashes.
www.mayoclinic.com/health/menopause/DS00119

National Center for Complementary and Alternative Medicine, National Institutes of Health

This government-sponsored site provides research-based information on complementary and alternative therapies for professionals and consumers. It covers an extensive list of treatments under the section, Topics A-Z.
http://nccam.nih.gov/

North American Menopause Society (NAMS)

The Web site of this organization has information on hot flashes. On the home page you will find information under the Ask the Experts section. If you click on For Consumers you will find more information, including in the downloadable Menopause Guidebook.
www.menopause.org/

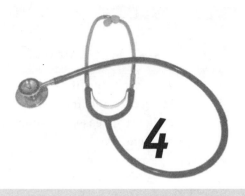

4

Sleep Disturbances: How Do I Get Some Rest?

I used to be such a deep sleeper. My head would hit the pillow and I'd be out till morning. Once, when I was a kid, we had a burglar in our bedroom and I slept through my sister screaming and my father chasing him off with a baseball bat. They woke me up when the police got there. Since menopause, forget it. I start to fall asleep okay and then, bam! Wide awake, sometimes for hours.   KRISTINE

Sleeping? What's that? What I do at night is something other than sleeping. It changed the moment I hit menopause. I haven't slept well since.   FRAN

Adults need seven to nine hours of sleep each night. Chronic insomnia has a significant negative impact on a person's quality of life. Not only does lack of sleep result in reduced productivity and irritability, it can have serious health consequences including depression, increased susceptibility to illness, increased risk of heart disease, and increased likelihood of having a serious accident.

Forty percent of menopausal women report sleeping problems; however, this is the same percentage as the population in general, so problems may not be related to menopause at all. A number of studies have found that postmenopausal women actually have as good or better sleep than the population in general. Sleep studies indicate that after menopause it is sleep efficiency that suffers, not our total sleep time. Sleep efficiency is the percentage of time in bed that is spent in sleep. After menopause it takes longer to fall asleep and less time is spent in restorative deep sleep (slow wave sleep). Because they spend a greater part of the time in light sleep, menopausal women are more sensitive to noise and other disturbances, and hence awaken more easily. Poor sleep efficiency means that even if the total amount of time you sleep during the night doesn't change, it feels like you're sleeping less.

Two symptoms related to menopause have been found to be associated with poor sleep in perimenopausal and postmenopausal women—hot flashes and anxiety. Women with these symptoms are more likely to have difficulty in getting to sleep and are more likely to report poor sleep. Awakenings from hot flashes generally happen only in the first half of the night though, not during the second half when you spend most of the time in rapid eye movement (REM) sleep. REM sleep suppresses thermoregulation and it may be suppressing hot flashes along with it. So once you are in a sound sleep hot flashes are not likely to wake you up. Anxiety is also more likely to cause difficulty in getting to sleep rather than cause awakenings during the night.

Much of the trouble sleeping encountered during the menopausal transition and postmenopause are actually related to two primary sleep disorders, restless legs syndrome (RLS) and sleep apnea. Studies have found that perimenopausal and postmenopausal women have higher rates of these disorders than

Sleep: A Primer

The Five Stages of Sleep

During sleep our brain repeatedly cycles through five stages. The stage is determined by the type of brain waves present. When we are awake our brain patterns exhibit beta waves when we are active and alpha waves when we are relaxed. When we are asleep our brain patterns exhibit slower theta and delta waves. Each cycle lasts an average of an hour and a half to two hours. As the night progresses, the time we spend in each deep sleep cycle, Stages 3 and 4, shortens and the REM stage lengthens.

- Stage 1: This stage is a gradual transition from relaxed wakefulness to sleep. Muscle activity slows down. Sleep is light and we are easily awakened. This stage is characterized by slow theta waves. It lasts only about 5 to 10 minutes.
- Stage 2: Theta waves continue during this stage. What differentiates it from Stage 1 are periodic bursts of rapid brain waves called sleep spindles and taller brain waves called K waves. Sleep continues to be light in this stage. In fact, if we are awakened during Stage 1 or 2 we may not even realize we had been asleep at all. This stage lasts about 20 minutes.
- Stage 3: Extremely slow brain waves called deltas begin to appear along with faster smaller waves. This stage is the transition between light sleep and deep sleep.
- Stage 4: Brain waves are almost all extremely slow delta waves. This is a very deep sleep and lasts about 30 minutes.

  - Stages 3 and 4 are deep sleep and it is difficult to awaken someone during this part of the sleep cycle. If you are awakened during this stage you'll feel disoriented and groggy for a few minutes.
  - At this point the stages reverse themselves. We quickly cycle back through Stages 4, 3, 2, 1 and then go immediately into the next stage—REM.

- REM Stage: This is the dream phase of sleep. During the REM stage breathing becomes rapid and shallow, heart rate increases, blood pressure rises, eyes moves rapidly in multiple directions, and arms and legs become temporarily paralyzed (so we don't act out our dreams).

Circadian rhythm

We all have an internal 24-hour biological clock that regulates waking and sleeping. The circadian clock is a small bundle of cells located in the hypothalamus. It responds to visual clues about light and dark. Certain cells in the retina of the eye, photosensitive ganglion cells, respond to light by sending signals to the pineal gland, which controls the release of melatonin. Darkness increases melatonin production while light decreases it to almost nil.

What Nurses Know...

Stat Facts

- *Forty percent of menopausal women report getting a good night's sleep every night or almost every night. This is the same as the percentage of women in general.*

- *Fifty to seventy million American adults suffer from chronic sleep problems.*

- *Twenty million Americans suffer from occasional sleeping problems.*

- *Eighteen million Americans suffer from sleep apnea and 10 million of them do not know it.*

- *Approximately 10 percent of all people have RLS.*

- *There are currently 70 different recognized sleeping disorders.*

other women. During one recent study, RLS and apnea, rather than hot flashes, caused most of the sleep problems observed. The occurrence of these disorders increases with aging, as well, so it is unclear how much of the problem is directly related to menopause and how much is the result of other age-related changes.

When you are staring at the alarm clock advancing steadily toward morning, you probably don't care if it is menopause or age that is keeping you awake. You just want to sleep. However, don't assume your sleep problems are just another menopausal annoyance to be endured. It is important to determine what is causing your sleeping problems so you can take the correct actions to resolve them and avoid long-term health consequences.

What Nurses Know...

Keep a sleep diary. It will help you see sleeping patterns and behaviors that may be contributing to sleeping difficulty. It is also an important part of a sleep evaluation. Record the following for two weeks:

- *Exercise done that day*

- *Caffeine intake and times*

- *Medication taken and times*

- *Alcohol use that day*

- *Activities during the hour before going to bed*

- *Food or drinks consumed before sleep and times*

- *Time you went to bed*

- *How long it took to fall asleep*

- *How often during the night you woke up and how long you were awake each time*

- *Noise or other disturbances*

- *Dreams*

- *Time you wake up*

- *How you feel when you wake up*

Restless Legs Syndrome

RLS is a neurological condition that causes unpleasant sensations in the legs when you're at rest, along with an irresistible urge to move your legs to try to relieve the sensations. The sensations are described as crawling, tingling, pulling, or creeping deep inside the legs. They are distressing but not painful. Most often the symptoms are in both legs from the knee to the ankle, though occasionally it affects only one leg or other parts of the body, such as the thighs or arms. Walking, kicking, or other leg movements improve the symptoms. There are different severity levels of RLS, from mild infrequent episodes that cause little problems to frequent severe episodes that have a major negative impact on the person's quality of life.

The cause of RLS is unknown. In 40 to 60 percent of cases that develop before the age of 40 there is a family history, indicating that there is a genetic component involved. This is less likely in people who develop the condition after the age of 50, however, when some kind of neurological problem is more likely the underlying factor.

A hallmark of the condition is that the symptoms start when you relax, and the more relaxed you are the more likely it is the symptoms will start. This makes falling asleep very difficult, especially since symptoms tend also to be worse at night. RLS can cause serious sleep deprivation for people who have moderate to severe cases.

About 80 percent of people with RLS also have another primary sleep disorder, periodic limb movements of sleep (PLMS). This condition causes periodic repetitive leg movements that occur every 20 to 40 seconds, mostly during sleep stages 1 and 2. The occurrence of PLMS gets more common as we get older. It is estimated that PLMS

• •

Criteria for Diagnosis of RLS

According to the International Restless Legs Syndrome Study Group, the four criteria for diagnosis of RLS are:

1. An urge to move, usually due to uncomfortable sensations that occur primarily in the legs
2. Motor restlessness, expressed as activity, that relieves the urge to move
3. Worsening of symptoms by relaxation
4. Variability over the course of the day–night cycle, with symptoms worse in the evening and early in the night.

International Restless Legs Syndrome Study Group (2006), RLS Information
www.irlssg.org/rlsinformation.html

occurs in five percent of people between the ages of 30 and 50 but increases to about 40 percent of people over 65 years of age.

TREATMENT OF RESTLESS LEGS SYNDROME

If you are diagnosed with RLS, you and your health care provider need to determine the best treatment approach for you depending on your particular symptoms and their frequency and severity. The first thing is to have a serum ferritin level done; this is a blood test to check your iron level. There is a high rate of iron deficiency in people with RLS. If your iron level is low, you can take oral iron supplements. It has been found that correcting iron deficiency greatly improved or even completely resolved RLS in people with iron deficiency.

• •

Alert

Do not take iron supplements without first having your blood level checked. It could be dangerous—too much iron in the blood can cause damage to the liver and heart. And studies found that oral iron supplementation made no difference in RLS symptoms in people with normal iron levels.

What Nurses Know...

The most effective way to take iron supplements is on an empty stomach. However, iron supplements can cause gastrointestinal side effects including nausea, vomiting, diarrhea, and constipation. Taking the iron in smaller divided doses and taking it with food will help decrease these side effects. Do not take it with milk, though; it will decrease absorption even more. Enteric-coated iron tablets are better tolerated but they are not as well absorbed.

Ask your health care provider about taking your iron supplements with vitamin C if you are not already doing this. It will improve absorption.

Iron supplements will also cause your stools to be dark or black.

Your health care provider should be checking your blood iron levels every three months to monitor the effectiveness of the supplementation and to make sure your levels don't get too high.

There are a number of different medications used to treat RLS. If your symptoms occur every night, then you will want to consider a medication that is taken daily. Otherwise you can choose a medication that acts quickly and take it when symptoms start or shortly before situations that usually cause symptoms, before a long car ride for instance. Some medications may be addictive or cause what is known as augmentation—over time symptoms begin to occur earlier and earlier in the day. Ask your health care provider about these side effects when deciding on treatment. Following is a list of the types of medications commonly used to treat RLS.

Medications for Treatment of RLS

- *Dopaminergic Medications*—these are drugs used primarily in the treatment of Parkinson's disease. Side effects include nausea and vomiting, hallucinations, and drop in blood pressure when rising after lying down or from a seated or crouched position. Can cause augmentation of symptoms.
- *Sedative–Hypnotic Medications*—these are drugs used primarily in the treatment of anxiety. Side effects include sedation and impaired mental functioning. You can build up a tolerance for these drugs, needing higher and higher doses over time to get the same effect. Can also be addictive.
- *Antiepileptic Medications*—these are drugs used primarily in the treatment of seizure disorders. Side effects include sedation, dizziness, fatigue, and motor incoordination.
- *Opiates*—these are drugs used primarily for pain relief. Side effects include sedation, nausea, vomiting, and constipation. Can be addictive.

Sleep Apnea

Sleep apnea, also called sleep disordered breathing, is a condition in which a person has repeated pauses in his or her breathing during sleep. People with sleep apnea are not aware of the apnea or the sleep disruption that accompanies it. It can range from mild infrequent pauses to severe interruptions that result in repeated drops in the oxygen supply your body is getting.

Sleep apnea is usually caused by an obstructed airway. Normally during sleep the muscles of the throat relax but the upper throat stays open enough to allow air flow into the lungs. In obstructive sleep apnea (OSA) the upper part of the throat closes off completely or almost completely, blocking air from getting to the lungs and causing a brief spell of stalled breathing. The person makes a sudden attempt to breathe, awakening slightly each time. Someone with OSA usually has loud snoring interrupted by periods of silence when their breathing pauses, then they inhale with a gasp and loud snort and breathing and snoring starts in again. This may happen as few as 10 times to as many as 100 times a night.

There is a significantly higher rate of sleep apnea in women during the menopausal transition and in the postmenopausal years. Studies also indicate that OSA is more severe in postmenopausal women. If you have daytime sleepiness or poor sleep, talk to your health care provider about having a sleep study done. OSA is harmful to your health; it can result in heart arrhythmias, high blood pressure, heart disease, and stroke. Sleep deprivation can lead you to fall asleep in situations that put you at risk, like behind the wheel of a car, for example. People with OSA are six times more likely to be involved in automobile accidents than those who don't have OSA.

TREATMENT OF OBSTRUCTIVE SLEEP APNEA

Obesity is a reversible cause of OSA and losing weight will often correct the problem. Otherwise, continuous positive airway pressure (CPAP) is the first-line treatment for OSA. CPAP is a device that delivers air under slight pressure through a tight-fitting mask you wear over your nose during sleep. The increased pressure keeps

Signs and Symptoms of OSA

If someone shares your sleeping space, ask them if they have observed the first three symptoms, as you will not be aware of them. If you sleep alone and suspect you may have OSA based on other symptoms, talk to your provider about having a sleep study done.

- *Loud snoring*
- *Periods of apnea during sleep*
- *Restless sleep*
- *Daytime sleepiness*
- *Wake up feeling tired*
- *Morning headaches*
- *Lethargic feeling*
- *Poor concentration*

the throat muscles open. There are also dental devices that change the position of the jaw, tongue, and soft palate to prevent blockage of the airway. Sleeping on your back tends to worsen sleep apnea, so changing to a side sleeping position can be helpful.

You should also have your health care provider check your thyroid function. Hypothyroid can be an underlying cause of OSA and treatment with thyroid replacement hormone can resolve OSA. There is no evidence to support the use of other medications in the treatment of OSA, including estrogen therapy. You should avoid alcohol, sleeping medications, and sedatives if you have OSA, as they will worsen apnea.

Getting a Good Night's Sleep

Check out any Web site or article on insomnia and you are bound to find advice about sleep hygiene. (Sleep hygiene simply means your bedtime and sleeping habits.) The American Academy of Sleep, however, concluded in a recent review that there isn't enough evidence to recommend sleep hygiene changes as a therapy for insomnia. This doesn't mean that it doesn't work. There just haven't been enough well done research studies that looked specifically at sleep hygiene to support its recommendation as a single therapy. Further research may find that it is effective and future recommendations can change.

In the meantime, you shouldn't ignore your sleep hygiene. Although it is not a cause of insomnia, it will worsen it. Making changes in your bedtime habits can help improve sleep and is often used in combination with other therapies. There are no potential harmful effects and it's free. It can make a difference on an individual basis. So it is worthwhile trying the changes suggested below before more costly measures and certainly before resorting to medications, which always carry some risk.

Sleep Hygiene

The best thing you can do to improve sleep hygiene is to develop a bedtime routine and follow it every night. You want to train your mind and body to associate certain activities and certain places—the bed and bedroom—with sleep. The first rule is to go to bed the same time every night and wake up the same time every morning, including nonwork days. Wind down about 30 to 60 minutes before bedtime. Turn off the television and computer. Take a warm bath. Meditate. Do gentle yoga. Read a book, but not a horror novel or one that is intellectually demanding—the key is to relax and soothe your mind, not stimulate it.

Another key is to reserve your bed for two things only—sleep and sex. Do not read, watch television, eat or use your laptop in bed. Sleep and sex only.

You want to limit the amount of time you spend awake in bed. If you don't fall asleep after 20 minutes, get out of bed. Do something relaxing like reading, gentle yoga, or listening to music. Do not watch television, get on the Internet, or work. When you feel sleepy, go back to bed. If you're still awake after another 20 minutes—get up and do it again.

Following are other ways to improve your sleep hygiene.

- A light bedtime snack, preferably one high in carbohydrates, can be helpful, but avoid large or fatty meals close to bedtime.

Gravity aids digestion and lying down soon after eating can lead to indigestion that will disrupt sleep. Fatty foods take longer to digest.

- Avoid drinking too many fluids at night so you won't need to wake up to go to the bathroom.
- Avoid caffeine four hours before bed, or even better, none after lunchtime.
- No nightcaps! Alcohol may relax you and make you sleepy initially but it keeps you in sleep Stages 1 and 2 and you won't get important restorative sleep. Ideally, you should not have alcohol within six hours of bedtime.
- Do not nap during the day. If you must nap limit it to 20 minutes before three o'clock in the afternoon and at least six hours before bedtime.
- Sleep in the dark; the darker the better. If you can block out any source of light, including the face of your alarm clocks, do so.
- Keep the temperature of the room cool. Those of you having hot flashes probably already do this.
- Do everything you can to ensure a quiet environment.

What Nurses Know ...

Nursing is an around-the-clock job, so many nurses have to learn to sleep when the rest of their part of the world is awake and active—and making noise. One trick they use frequently is turning on a fan for white noise. White noise is noise that has a combination of all the different frequencies of sound. It prevents your brain from focusing in on any one sound, effectively canceling out all of them. You can buy white noise machines, but an inexpensive fan is likely to work just as well.

Behavioral Treatments

There are a number of treatments that research has shown to be effective and are recommended by the American Academy of Sleep. They are called cognitive behavioral therapy (CBT) and include stimulus control therapy, relaxation training, sleep restriction therapy, biofeedback, and paradoxical intention. Sleep hygiene is often used in conjunction with one or more of these techniques.

Behavioral treatment is more effective than sleep medication. It works in 70 to 80 percent of people who try it. You have to be willing to give it time though; it will take longer to see results than popping a pill does. But once you start sleeping better the results will last.

Following is a brief description of effective CBT techniques. Most of these therapies need to be done with guidance from a sleep therapist or someone trained in the technique. Talk to your health care provider or contact a sleep center or sleep specialist. (See Resources at the end of this chapter for help in finding a sleep center or sleep specialist.)

Stimulus Control Therapy–the goal of this therapy is to reestablish the association of bed with sleep and replace the negative response to bedtime with positive expectations of sleep.

Relaxation Training–this therapy involves using relaxation techniques, such as progressive muscle relaxation, to relieve body tension and intrusive thoughts at bedtime.

Sleep Restriction Therapy–limits the time spent in bed to the time spent sleeping. You take the average number of hours you actually spend sleeping a night and only allow yourself to be in bed for that amount of time. When you are sleeping throughout the time spent in bed, you gradually increase the time in bed until you are sleeping seven or eight hours a night.

Biofeedback–uses feedback to teach you to control certain body functions, like muscle control, to increase relaxation at bedtime.

Paradoxical Intention–relieves sleep "performance anxiety" at bedtime by teaching you to try staying awake rather than falling asleep.

Sleep Medications

There are a number of different types of medications used for sleep, both those available over the counter (OTC) and those requiring a prescription. All carry risks and should only be used after behavioral therapies have been tried unsuccessfully. The primary active ingredients in OTC sleeping medications are antihistamines. There are four types of prescription medications used for treating insomnia: benzodiazepines, nonbenzodiazepines, antidepressants, and melatonin receptor agonists.

OVER-THE-COUNTER SLEEP MEDICATIONS

Antihistamines are the primary active ingredients in OTC sleep medications. Antihistamines are generally used for

What Nurses Know...

Use drugs for sleeping problems only as a last resort. They always carry some risk and the risks increase as we age. When we are older we no longer metabolize many drugs as effectively as we did when we were younger, which can result in more severe side effects, oversedation, confusion, and impaired daytime functioning. Sedatives are a big culprit in falls that lead to hip fractures in the elderly. Even if you are still relatively young, you don't want to develop a habit of depending on sleep medications that will follow you into old age.

the treatment of allergies and cold symptoms like a stuffy or runny nose. The antihistamine most commonly used for sleep is diphenhydramine (Benadryl). You are probably familiar with diphenhydramine, and if you have ever taken it for a cold or allergies you are probably also familiar with one of its major side effects, drowsiness. It is this side effect that makes it and other antihistamines useful as a sleep medication. The other common antihistamine used for sleep is doxylamine (Unisom). Both these medications are used alone and in combination with other medications. They are often combined with acetaminophen (Tylenol), pseudoephedrine, and dextromethorphan in cold relief products.

Though many people use antihistamines regularly for sleep, there is little evidence to support their use as a treatment for insomnia. Research has found that antihistamines cause daytime sleepiness and impair your ability to function without real improvement in nighttime sleep. There is also some evidence that any benefit is greatly reduced after a few days.

Antihistamines dry up secretions that cause the runny nose and watery eyes associated with allergies. This drying effect is behind another common side effect, dry mouth. Drinking plenty of fluids during the day, chewing sugarless gum, and sucking on hard candy can help.

If you are taking antihistamines for sleep or think they may be a good option for you, talk to your health care provider about it. Antihistamines can interact with other medications and may

Alert

Be aware of all the ingredients in any OTC medication you are taking. Read the labels carefully for all active ingredients. Otherwise you can overdose by mistake. For example, you have a cold and decide to take Vicks NyQuil D at bedtime in addition to Unisom for sleep, not realizing they both contain doxylamine. Another common ingredient in sleep aids and cold medicines is acetaminophen (Tylenol), which can cause serious and even fatal liver failure in cases of overdosage.

What Nurses Know...

Do not be lulled into a false sense of security when taking OTC medications. They are not risk-free and can cause serious problems when not taken as directed. They may also interact with other medications you are on. Read labels carefully and make sure your health care provider is aware of all OTC medicine you are taking.

be contraindicated if you have certain health problems, such as asthma, emphysema, and glaucoma.

PRESCRIPTION MEDICATIONS

There are four types of prescription medications used to treat insomnia: benzodiazepines, nonbenzodiazepines, antidepressants, and the newcomer on the scene, melatonin receptor agonists. The first three have the potential for serious side effects, whereas melatonin receptor agonists currently appear to have few side effects. However, it is a newer medication and more research is needed, especially on long-term use.

Before deciding to take prescription medications to treat your insomnia, think about this: Their effect is very small. An analysis that looked at over 100 studies of benzodiazepines, nonbenzodiazepines, and antidepressants for sleep found that people who used them got to sleep at most 13 minutes sooner and stayed asleep only 11 minutes longer during the night. Ask yourself, are these small improvements worth the risks?

Benzodiazepines Benzodiazepines have many uses and are widely prescribed. Along with treating insomnia, they are used to treat anxiety, muscle spasms, and to prevent seizures. Benzodiazepines can be divided into two groups: short-acting benzodiazepines and long-acting benzodiazepines. Both are used in the treatment of insomnia. The short-acting benzodiaz-epines clear the body in a short period of time and are usually the choice if you have difficulty in falling asleep but no symptoms of anxiety. Long-acting benzodiazepines, which remain in the body a long time, are usually the choice if you have both problems sleeping at night and anxiety during the day.

There are a number of significant problems in using benzodi-azepines for sleep. Tolerance and addiction are two of the major ones. When you develop tolerance to a drug, you must continu-ally increase your dose in order to keep getting the same effect. Unfortunately, tolerance to the sleep effects of benzodiazepines develops very quickly when you take them regularly. Tolerance is a big factor in the potential for addiction to benzodiazepines.

Other problems include daytime sleepiness, memory prob-lems, dizziness, increased risk of falls, and car accidents. In studies of the effect of benzodiazepines on driving it was found that taking benzodiazepines at bedtime significantly impaired driving ability the next morning and sometimes even in the afternoon.

Benzodiazepines should *only be used intermittently for short-term relief* of insomnia. If you have been taking benzodiazepines

What Nurses Know...

The half-life of a drug is important in determining how long its effects will last. Half-life is the amount of time it takes for half of the drug to be cleared from your system. The longer the half-life, the longer the drug, and its effects, lasts in your system. Sometimes a long half-life is a good thing—it's a lot easier to take an antibiotic once a day rather than every four hours. But when you take a sleep-ing pill, you really don't want it still active in your system when it's time to wake up eight hours later.

What Nurses Know...

Take a holiday! A drug holiday that is. One strategy that can help prevent tolerance and lower the risk of side effects is to regularly schedule time off from a medication. This is known as a drug holiday *and is often used with people who take certain medications on a long-term, continual basis.*

for more than a few months, talk to your health care provider about other alternatives, like CBT. Do not stop benzodiazepines abruptly. You must taper off the medication gradually if you've been taking them regularly, otherwise you can experience withdrawal symptoms and worsening of your insomnia.

Commonly Prescribed Benzodiazepines

Short acting
Estazolam (Prosom)
Flurazepam (Dalmane)
Triazolam (Halcion)
Temazepam (Restoril)

Long acting
Alprazolam (Xanax)
Diazepam (Valium)
Lorazepam (Ativan)
Oxazepam (Serax)
Clonazepam (Klonopin)

Notice that all the generic names end with *lam* or *pam*? Though not all benzodiazepine drug names end with these suffixes, most do. So if a drug's name ends in *lam* or *pam*, then you know the drug is a benzodiazepine.

Nonbenzodiazepines   Medications in this class of sleeping drugs, also called benzodiazepine-like, are similar to benzodiazepines in the way they work. However, they have some important advantages over the older benzodiazepines. First, they are much less likely to cause addiction or tolerance. Second, they have a shorter half-life so you shouldn't wake up groggy or have effects lasting into the day. In fact, studies have found that, unlike benzodiazepines, driving is not impaired the next morning when the medication is taken at bedtime (though if you take it in the middle of the night, there may be some impairment in the morning).

One problem that has arisen with nonbenzodiazepines, though, are reports of bizarre sleep activities during the night. People have engaged in all kinds of complex behaviors in their sleep, such as preparing meals or driving a car. There have been reports of violent behavior as well. These events are relatively rare but must be considered in your decision to use these medications because they create a real safety risk for you and others.

Commonly Prescribed Nonbenzodiazepines

Zolpidem (Ambien)
Zaleplon (Sonata)
Eszopiclone (Lunesta)

Melatonin and Melatonin Receptor Agonists   Melatonin is a hormone produced deep in our brain in the pineal gland, that helps regulate the circadian rhythm and sleep and wake cycles. Production rises as evening progresses, stays high through the night, and drops off in the morning. Darkness increases production of melatonin and light suppresses it. Melatonin levels are highest at bedtime. Sleeping in absolute darkness helps maintain a high melatonin level.

As we get older we produce less melatonin, which is thought to play a role in the increase in sleeping problems as we age. It has also been found that decreasing levels of melatonin actually play a role in the onset of menopause. Research is now looking into what happens when women receive regular doses of melatonin during the menopausal transition and after menopause.

Melatonin supplements can help with sleep problems. There has been some research that shows that melatonin supplements help you fall asleep faster and stay asleep longer during the night. Further studies need to be done, but at this time there appears to be little risk of side effects with short-term use. It has been recommended for short-term use in women during perimenopause and postmenopause.

Melatonin receptor agonists are a new class of medication that bind to the same receptors in the brain that melatonin does, mimicking its actions. At present there is only one melatonin receptor agonist that has been approved by the Food and Drug Administration, ramelteon (Rozerem). In studies, people who took ramelteon got to sleep faster and had better sleep efficiency. There were few side effects, with headache the most common. Melatonin receptor agonists have a much longer half-life than melatonin supplements, which means they may be better in improving overall sleep time and sleep efficiency.

NATURAL PRODUCTS

Melatonin supplements are the most commonly used natural product for insomnia and the one with the most research on its use. Another natural product is the herb valerian. Valerian has been used for a long time for sleep problems and anxiety. There is very little research on its effectiveness, however. A few studies have shown it to be helpful for insomnia. It can cause headaches, dizziness, and upset stomach, and sometimes you will wake up feeling tired the morning after taking it. Do not take valerian if you are taking benzodiazepines or other antidepressant or anti-anxiety medications. Doing so can cause a dangerous overdose. Always include any natural products on the medication list you give to your health care provider.

And to All a Goodnight...

The more we learn about sleep the more it becomes apparent that it is vital for good health and happiness. Try the measures outlined earlier and talk to your health care provider about any symptoms that may indicate the presence of sleep apnea or RLS. Don't accept insomnia as an inevitable consequence of menopause.

Resources

American Academy of Sleep Medicine
The Web site for this organization has a Patients and Public site, a directory of sleep centers and labs, and a list of certified sleep medicine specialists.
www.aasmnet.org

MedlinePlus
Sleep Disorders
This National Institutes of Health Web site offers links to a wide range of information and materials on insomnia.
www.nlm.nih.gov/medlineplus/sleepdisorders.html

Restless Legs Syndrome Foundation
The Web site of this nonprofit organization provides information and a community chat room for those who suffer with RLS. It also maintains a directory of health care providers who specialize in RLS.
www.rls.org

American Sleep Apnea Association
The Web site of this nonprofit organization provides information, links to other resources, and information on support groups throughout the United States.
www.sleepapnea.org

Sexuality

I have noticed decreased sex drive but not decreased desire. I have also registered a feeling of no longer being sexually viable—not in my primary relationship but in the world. I no longer have "it." This can really take a person by surprise; there is no culturally sanctioned mourning for it. And it's a real loss. JOYCE

Intercourse just wasn't going to happen. It wasn't that I didn't want to have sex, it was just too painful! I didn't talk to my gyn for about six months. I didn't really see it as a problem at first because we were still enjoying sex— you just do other things! My husband was very good about it. In fact, one night he said, "Why don't you go to the doctor?" But it was because he was worried something was wrong. Ironically, I had just made an appointment that day. SUSAN

I don't have to use Astroglide! No pain or dryness or anything.
No real change in libido. At least nothing that changed after
menopause. I don't have the same level of desire as I used to
but it was a slow process. I think a lot of it has to do with
life. If I wasn't married maybe it'd be different. You know, it's
kind of like, been there done that after 30 years with the same
man. And then there's all the stuff going on with the kids, and
your job, and an aging mother. It's a lot.   LIZ

Almost all of the women who are perimenopausal or beyond experienced the sexual revolution of the 1960s. We are the first wave of post-birth control pill and women's liberation women. Most of us have spent our adult lives expecting sex to be joyful, uninhibited, and reciprocal. There is no reason we should not expect anything less now.

It is true that as the menopausal transition progresses sexual desire and satisfaction decrease for many women. It's important to keep things in perspective, however. For instance; take a look at the results of a recent study that looked at the changes in sexual functioning of over 17,000 women across the United States as they transitioned through menopause. Even though they found that overall sexual desire decreased over the menopausal transition and into postmenopause, 84 percent of women in late perimenopause reported feeling sexual desire at least once or twice a month and 46 percent of them desired sex at least once a week. After menopause 76 percent of the women reported sexual desire at least once or twice a month with 35 percent of them reporting it at least once a week. Even more encouraging, the level of arousal and physical pleasure were not related to menopause at all.

It's important to keep in mind that there are many things that affect your sexual functioning during these years other than hormonal changes related to menopause. The quality of your relationship, the availability of a partner, your overall health, your state of mind, and your attitudes about aging are all related to level of sexual desire and satisfaction. In fact, most studies show

What Nurses Know . . .

Changes in your level of sexual desire and response are only a problem if they cause you distress. Do not judge your sexuality against other people's ideas of what is "normal" at any age. There is only one "should" when it comes to sex—you should feel good about your sexual life, however active or inactive you choose it to be.

that these are more often the cause of sexual problems during perimenopause and afterward, not hormones.

In fact, the factor that had the most impact on a women's sexual functioning in the above study was the importance of sex. Women who rated sex as quite important or extremely important wanted sex more, had it more often, and enjoyed it more when they did. So, you see, it is really up to you. If a satisfying sex life is important to you, you can make it happen.

Understanding what to expect during perimenopause and after menopause is important to enjoying your sexuality to the fullest during this period of your life. There are many options available to address the physical changes that happen during the menopausal transition. Keep in mind that paying attention to your emotional health and your relationships is as important as any physical factor.

Hormones and Sex

Estrogen and testosterone are the two primary hormones involved in women's sexuality. Estrogen primarily acts on the reproductive organs themselves while testosterone is thought to be responsible for desire and arousal.

Estrogen maintains normal blood flow to the genitalia. Blood flow to genitalia increases during sexual response, swelling the clitoris and lubricating the vagina. Estrogen maintains the elasticity of the vagina, allowing for penetration. It also plays a role in sensory perception in the outer portion of the vagina.

It is widely reported that testosterone plays a role in sexual desire and response in women, yet how is not understood and there is no scientific evidence to support this. In fact, in the few studies that compared the level of testosterone in a woman's blood (naturally, without taking testosterone) and her level of sexual desire, most found no connection. Yet numerous studies do show that treatment with testosterone improves sexual desire and response in women.

Sex, Your Vagina, and Menopause

Perimenopause brings a number of changes to the genitalia. Vaginal atrophy, also called urogenital atrophy, is the biggest and has important implications for your sexual health.

Up to 40 percent of postmenopausal women report symptoms of vaginal atrophy. Symptoms are due to lack of estrogen and severity is related to the amount of estrogen present; the less estrogen the more severe the symptoms. Before menopause the walls of the vagina are rugated, meaning they are corrugated with ridges that fold onto themselves. This allows the vagina to expand without discomfort or tearing. As you progress through menopause, estrogen levels fall, the rugae smooth out, and the walls become less elastic. The vaginal lining becomes dry and thin. There are less vaginal secretions, so lubrication decreases as well.

The opening into the vagina, the introitus, begins to narrow early in perimenopause in many women. There is actually more narrowing in the outer portion of the vagina than further up. This is because the outer parts of the vagina are much more sensitive to estrogen and so have more dramatic changes when estrogen levels fall. Narrowing of the introitus, along with the thinning and drying vaginal tissues, is a primary cause of painful sexual intercourse (dyspareunia). It also makes your gynecological pelvic examination and Pap smear difficult and painful.

Vaginal pH balance changes as well. The term *pH* refers to the acidity or alkalinity of a solution. For optimal vaginal health, secretions should be acidic. The acidic environment of the vagina promotes the growth of protective organisms, especially lactobacillus. These organisms prevent the growth of unwanted bacteria, like yeast (*Candida*). As estrogen levels decrease during perimenopause, vaginal pH rises, becoming less acidic, and you become more prone to vaginal infections.

All of these changes can progress to a condition called atrophic vaginitis. It is atrophic vaginitis that causes symptoms of dryness, itching, burning, and painful intercourse. These symptoms resolve on their own in about half of women. It is not clear

What Nurses Know . . .

pH is measured on a scale of 0 to 14. The lower the pH, the more acidic a solution is. The higher the pH, the more alkaline, or base, the solution is. When a solution is in the middle, having a value of 7, it is neutral, neither acidic nor alkaline. Optimal vaginal pH, one that will keep unwanted bacteria in check, is from 3.5 to 4.5. During perimenopause your vaginal pH rises into the 5.0 to 6.5 range and after menopause will range from 6.0 to 7.5.

Vaginal infections will also cause the pH to rise. Your health care provider may check the pH as part of an examination to rule out certain vaginal infections. This test becomes less predictive once you are in perimenopause, as a higher vaginal pH may be a normal finding.

why this happens. It may be that women adjust to the changes and are no longer bothered by them or their sexual activity changes. Or it may be that the vaginal tissue adapts as hormonal changes level off over time.

There are things you can do to alleviate symptoms and prevent atrophic vaginitis. It is important to do so for a number of reasons. Atrophic vaginitis can have a major impact on your quality of life. It can cause significant discomfort; it increases your risk for vaginal and urinary tract infections; it makes you more vulnerable to sexually transmitted infections (STIs) if you are sexually active; and vaginal symptoms are a primary cause of lower arousal, decreased emotional satisfaction, and less physical pleasure with sex.

Strategies

SEX

We set a time for sex, put it on the schedule so it's a special time just for us and for that. We try for the afternoon since

What Nurses Know . . .

Do not assume that all vaginal symptoms are related to menopausal changes. Itching, burning, and painful intercourse can all be indications of conditions needing treatment, usually vaginal or urinary tract infections. Yeast infections especially like the higher pH environment that comes with menopause. If you have a new onset of symptoms or worsening of existing symptoms, follow up with your health care provider.

What Nurses Know...

Talk to your health care provider about sexual problems that are causing you distress. It is not unusual to feel embarrassed bringing up the topic. You can start by bringing up something you have read in this chapter to break the ice. The hardest part is getting the conversation started, but once you get past that you may be surprised how easily the discussion goes. If your health care provider seems uncomfortable or doesn't take your concerns seriously, then find someone who does. Sexual distress has a major impact on your quality of life and you deserve to have it addressed like any other health problem.

we have the most energy then. Recently we started sunbathing nude and that can really get the juices going!   FRAN

I haven't had a partner since I hit menopause and sometimes I worry what will happen when I have sex again. Will it hurt too much? Will I even be able to do it? But for now I have a vibrator and I use it, often. Partly because I think it will keep me ready for when that next passionate affair comes along, but mostly because it just feels good!   KRISTINE

One of the best things you can do for ongoing sexual health is to have ongoing sex. Regular sexual activity is critical in maintaining optimum vaginal health. It helps prevent atrophic vaginitis, prevents loss of elasticity and narrowing of the vaginal opening, and increases lubrication. Studies indicate that women who are sexually active experience fewer symptoms of vaginal atrophy.

And sex begets sex. How sexually active you were in the past is a big factor in how active you are today. How active you are today will help determine how active you'll be in the future. Studies show that sexual activity levels tend to endure over time unless there is a major disruption, such as the loss of your partner or a major change in your health.

Don't count yourself out if you have no partner. Masturbation counts. Engaging in masturbation has much of the same positive effects on vaginal and sexual health. Masturbation has always been considered an important activity in helping women connect with their own sexuality and become more orgasmic. It is never too late to discover yourself sexually; it's not only enjoyable, it's good for you!

If you have not been sexually active for a long time and want to resume sexual intercourse you may need to prepare your vagina for penetration. This can be done with graded vaginal dilators. Vaginal dilators are smooth cylinders made of plastic or silicone that come in graduated sizes. Using a lubricant you insert one into your vagina for a short period of time, usually 15 minutes, beginning with the smallest one and gradually working up to the largest. You should use vaginal dilators under the guidance of a health care provider who can direct you on their proper use. They are usually used in combination with vaginal estrogen and pelvic muscle exercises. Graded vaginal dilators can also help when vaginal stenosis makes pelvic exams too painful for a woman to get recommended checkups and Pap smears.

MOISTURIZERS AND LUBRICANTS

Vaginal moisturizers help combat vaginal lining dryness. They are applied into the vagina with an applicator and are absorbed into the vaginal tissue. Most are supposed to last two or three days. One study found that a long-lasting moisturizer available over the counter (Replens) was similar to vaginal estrogen in relief of vaginal symptoms. It lowered vaginal pH as well. Some women find these products inconvenient and messy to use. You may have a discharge with use or leak some of the moisturizer that is not absorbed by the vagina. Vaginal moisturizers can be combined with other lubricants.

Using lubricants during sexual intercourse is another option. There are many lubricants available over the counter. Make sure that you choose one that is water-based and water-soluble, not oil- or petroleum-based. Oil- and petroleum-based lubricants increase your risk of vaginal infections since they tend to hold onto bacteria. They also damage condoms and diaphragms, making them less effective.

STAY HEALTHY

Your overall health is important to your sexual health. Studies consistently find that good health is good for your sex life. In a 2007 study of sexuality and health among 3,000 people in the United States from 57 to 85 years of age, it was found that people who reported being in good health were more likely to be sexually active and reported fewer sexual problems. Women who thought they were in excellent or very good health were more than three times as likely to be sexually active as those who thought their health was fair or poor. When over 2,000 women completed questionnaires on sexual activities and quality of life, women who reported greater sexual frequency were those who reported better health status.

A big part of good health is being physically active. Staying active has so many benefits, especially as we get older. People who are physically active have lower blood pressure, reduced risk of cardiovascular disease, greater muscle strength, and increased stamina. Add to that list—better sex. Women who are physically active report fewer vaginal symptoms and a more active sex life. Exercise also can make you look and feel better, both of which will enhance your feeling of sexuality.

For more information on health and fitness take a look at Chapter 10.

MIX IT UP

Sexual activity is not limited to intercourse. Intimacy doesn't have to end because penetration is no longer pleasurable. If painful

What Nurses Know...

A number of medications can decrease sexual desire and responsiveness. Talk to your health care provider if you are on any of the medications listed below. There may be alternatives or perhaps your dose can be adjusted.

- Benzodiazepines
- Antidepressants
- Cholesterol medications
- Cardiac medications
    - Beta blockers
    - Clonidine
    - Digoxin
- Dilantin
- Indomethacin (Indocin)
- Antihistamines
- Blood pressure medications
- Narcotics

intercourse is a problem you can't get past, then consider other ways to give and get sexual pleasure. Mutual masturbation and oral sex are two of the better known alternatives to intercourse. Buy a book on sex for some more ideas. There's the old classic, *The Joy of Sex*, as well as a number of books specifically for people over 40 or 50. Finding a position that gives you more control of thrusting and penetration depth can help ease painful intercourse.

Reclaiming your sexuality may be a matter of reigniting old fires or starting new ones. Give yourself the freedom to be adventurous. Change your foreplay routine. Share your fantasies. Read erotica together out loud. Try adding sex toys to your repertoire, or vaginal lubricants that are flavored or warm up on contact.

COUNSELING

Counseling can be helpful, especially when there are personal or relationship issues involved. Learning how to adapt to a changing relationship and sexual dynamics during these years is difficult. Many experts believe that some of the sexual problems blamed on menopause are actually long-standing issues that menopausal changes just unmasked.

Sometimes it can feel easier to just let things go along and accept the limitations of your sex life. But fighting for a satisfying sex life is worth it when intimacy is important to you. Counseling can help you explore underlying issues that may be the real barrier to a satisfying sex life. Couples counseling can be particularly helpful in a long-term relationship where one or the other may be carrying "baggage" picked up along the way.

Sex therapy is another option to give you the tools needed to recover and rediscover your sexuality. Seeing a sex therapist is similar to seeing any counselor. During the initial visit, the therapist will take a detailed history and then you and she or he will identify problems and decide on goals for the therapy. Treatment may include information and activities and exercises for you to do at home.

Sexual communication skills are often a big part of sex therapy. Learning to ask for what you want and letting your partner know what feels good and what doesn't becomes even more important during this time of changes.

Hormone Therapy

In this section we will talk about vaginal estrogen therapy (ET) and testosterone treatment. For a full discussion of ET, check out Chapters 7 and 8.

VAGINAL ESTROGEN

The good news is that very small amounts of topical estrogen can prevent or reverse atrophic vaginal changes. Vaginal estrogen has less risk of side effects than oral estrogen and may have better, and faster, results for vaginal symptoms. Very little of it is absorbed into your system. Improvement is usually seen two to four weeks after starting treatment.

Before beginning topical estrogen treatment your health care provider should do a history and physical examination to rule out other causes of vaginal symptoms. Bring a list of all medications you are taking, including over-the-counter drugs. Some, like antihistamines, may be contributing to dryness. Vaginal preparations come in creams, rings, and tablets. All of them are effective, so which you use is a matter of personal choice.

Creams   Vaginal estrogen creams (Estrace, Premarin Cream) usually have higher levels of estrogen than tablets. In fact, doses can be high enough to alleviate hot flashes for some women.

Using creams is easy. They come with an applicator, which you screw onto the tube of cream. You squeeze the cream into the applicator and then unscrew the applicator from the tube. Lying on your back you insert the applicator into your vagina and press the plunger, pushing the cream into your vagina. After removing the applicator, you wash it with soap and water and use it again.

Rings   Vaginal estrogen also comes in a flexible ring (Estring) about two inches in diameter. It is inserted into the upper part of the vagina where it releases estrogen slowly over three months. If you have vaginal stenosis or a shortened, narrow vagina, you may not be able to use the ring.

If you have ever used a diaphragm for birth control, you will be familiar with the insertion procedure. It is very easy. Press the sides of the ring together using your thumb and index finger and gently push it as far as you can up into the vagina, the farther the better. It will feel more comfortable and be less likely to fall out the farther back it is. Don't worry, you can't push it too far, it will only go as far as the cervix. If it feels uncomfortable, try pushing it farther back or remove it and try reinserting it. There should not be any discomfort when it is in place; you should not even be aware it is there. If you continue to have discomfort, remove it and follow up with your health care provider. You should also follow up if the ring falls out a lot, even when you place it far enough back.

Sometimes the ring may move or come out when you move your bowels, especially if you are constipated and need to strain. Rinse it off and reinsert it if this happens. If it happens repeatedly, you can just remove it before moving your bowels and reinsert it afterward.

You can engage in sexual intercourse with the ring in, but some women feel better removing it when they have sex.

Tablets Vaginal estrogen tablets (Vagifem) are packaged individually and attached to an applicator. You remove the applicator from the wrapper, stand with one leg on a chair and gently insert the applicator, with one finger on the plunger. Do not insert more than half the applicator into the vagina or push it in past the point of comfort. Press the applicator. You should hear a click, which indicates the tablet has been released. Remove the applicator and throw it away. If during insertion the tablet falls out of the applicator, don't try to reattach it; throw it and the applicator away.

TESTOSTERONE TREATMENT

Numerous studies have found that treatment with testosterone improves sexual desire and response in women who have problems with sexual function. These improvements were modest overall (average was about one additional sexual encounter a month) and usually only achieved at a dose that raised the testosterone level above what is normal for women naturally (which raises the risk of side effects). Also, to date, the research has looked only at testosterone combined with ET, so the effectiveness and safety of taking testosterone alone is not known. This raises concerns because testosterone treatment carries known side effects and risks.

Taking testosterone can cause acne and excessive growth of body and facial hair (hirsutism). More worrisome however are concerns about cardiovascular disease and breast cancer in women taking testosterone. Testosterone lowers high-density lipoproteins (the good cholesterol) and increases low-density lipoproteins, which can put you at increased risk of cardiovascular disease. A 2009 study found that postmenopausal women with higher levels of testosterone had triple the rate of heart disease and metabolic syndrome as postmenopausal women with lower testosterone levels. There is also an increased risk of liver disease, including cancer, when higher doses are used.

There is also a question of increased risk of breast cancer in women taking testosterone. Studies of women treated with testosterone/estrogen combination medications show an increased rate of breast cancer. Studies of testosterone taken alone are mixed, and more research is needed before the safety of taking it is known. With what we know now, if you or a family member has a history of breast cancer you are not a good candidate for testosterone treatment.

Currently, testosterone is not approved in the United States for treatment of sexual dysfunction in women during perimenopause or postmenopause. Testosterone patches for sexual dysfunction are approved in Europe and the United Kingdom. There is a combined estrogen–testosterone oral tablet, which is approved by the Food and Drug Administration (FDA) for treatment of hot flashes and night sweats only. However, it and other testosterone products are often prescribed off-label for women with low or absent sexual desire.

Remember, hormonal changes are not necessarily the culprit for sexual problems during and after the menopausal transition. Before deciding to try treatment with testosterone, with all the risks it entails, make sure you've addressed the other more likely causes of sexual dysfunction such as painful intercourse, other health problems, and relationship issues.

If, after addressing all of the above, lack of sexual desire and response is still a big problem, then a low dose of testosterone along with ET may be appropriate for a short period of time. As with any medications, you must weigh the risks against the benefits. This begins with a frank discussion with your health care provider. All of the following needs to be included in that discussion:

- How loss of sexual desire is affecting your quality of life
- Possible other factors that may be causing sexual problems
- What strategies you have already tried
- Personal or family history of heart disease
- Personal or family history of stroke
- Your lipid profile (results of blood tests for cholesterol levels)
- Personal or family history of breast cancer
- Recent research on testosterone treatment

The next step is a complete physical examination, including:

- Pelvic examination
- Breast examination and mammogram
- Blood tests
    - Lipid levels
    - Thyroid function
    - Complete blood count
    - Hormone levels
    - Liver function tests

After all of the above, you and your health care provider may decide that a *short-term* trial of testosterone treatment is appropriate for you. Generally, testosterone treatment will not be recommended for women with a history of breast cancer, liver disease, or cardiovascular disease.

Testosterone is usually prescribed in combination with estrogen. There is very little information about the effectiveness and safety of testosterone used alone, and it should not be prescribed without ET.

The most common form of testosterone prescribed for women are transdermal products. Transdermal products are those that are absorbed through the skin. This includes gels, creams, and ointments. Usually these are custom-compounded products. Use a compounding pharmacy recommended by your health care provider. (For more information on custom-compounding, take a look at Chapter 8.)

Testosterone also comes in a transdermal patch, but there are no patches available in the United States with doses that are low enough for women. In 2004, the FDA denied approval of a testosterone patch designed to treat lack of sexual desire and response in women (Intrinsa, a product of Procter & Gamble). They cited the minimal changes seen with its use (in studies, women who used it reported on average only one additional satisfying sexual event per month) and concerns about long-term safety as reasons for the denial. Do not try using part of a male testosterone patch; there is no way to adjust the dosage and you can end up with testosterone levels that are too high. Too much testosterone in women causes virilization; a deepening voice, increased muscle mass, and severe hirsutism or male-pattern baldness.

What Nurses Know ...

Money Matters

Health insurance may not cover medications when they are used off-label. Check with your health insurance plan before ordering medication. Custom-compounded hormone costs vary but usually range from $30 to $60 per hormone (some preparations contain multiple hormones) for a one month supply.

Alert

DO NOT buy testosterone products advertised on the Internet. There is no way of knowing what is in the product and what dose of testosterone you are getting. You can end up with a product that is either dangerous or useless!

The more promises made about a product, the less likely they are to be true. This holds true for any product. Remember what your mother told you—if it sounds too good to be true it probably is.

Testosterone can also be administered through an injection or in tablets that dissolve under your tongue. Both of these have a number of disadvantages and are usually not prescribed for women. The biggest problem is difficulty with accurate dosing at the lower doses needed for women. Others include pain with the injections and bad taste with the tablets.

What Nurses Know...

Always use topical medications as directed. When medication is applied to the skin or mucous membranes, some of it is absorbed into your system. If applied over a larger area of the body than for which it is intended, or applied more frequently than recommended, higher levels will be absorbed into the body, increasing the risk of side effects or an overdose.

Always wash your hands after applying topical or transdermal medications. There have been reports of children being exposed to testosterone through contact with someone being treated with transdermal testosterone. You should also cover the area where it is applied with clothing.

Your health care provider should monitor your response to testosterone treatment. This includes how well it is working for you and the presence of any side effects. It is a good idea to do blood tests after three months to recheck your lipid levels and liver function.

DEHYDROEPIANDROSTERONE

You may have heard about another hormone called dehydroepiandrosterone (DHEA). It is produced in the adrenal glands and is an early part of the production of testosterone and estrogen. There are reports that it will increase your sexual desire and response. Currently, there is no evidence to support this and little is known about long-term effects. Until further research is done, it is not recommended.

Birth Control

You probably know someone who got a big surprise when they discovered their missed periods were not due to perimenopause after all, but to a very unexpected pregnancy. Unfortunately, far too many women make the mistake of thinking they are home free when it comes to contraception once they miss a few periods. You can still get pregnant until you have reached menopause, and menopause is not confirmed until twelve months have passed without a period.

Pregnancy carries greater risk for both mother and infant after age 40; rates of gestational diabetes, cesarean delivery, birth defects, and premature delivery all increase. Unplanned pregnancy can result in delayed prenatal care and exposure to food and other substances harmful to a developing fetus.

There really isn't any birth control method that is not advised on the basis of perimenopause alone. It really comes down to personal choice, unless there are health conditions that rule out the use of certain methods. There is some concern about the use of medroxyprogesterone acetate (Depo-Provera), an injectable form of progesterone that is given every three months. Research indicates that its use may increase bone loss and increase your risk of osteoporosis.

If you have sexual intercourse infrequently, then you may want to consider one of the barrier methods, such as condoms or a diaphragm. You use it only when you need it and the side effects are few. They are not as effective as other methods, about 85 percent overall, though compliance, using it correctly *every* time, increases effectiveness.

Combined oral contraceptive pills (OCPs; containing estrogen and progestin) have many benefits for women during perimenopause, in addition to providing contraception. It can decrease hot flashes, regulate your menstrual period, reduce monthly bleeding, and decrease bone loss. OCPs lower your risk of ovarian cancer and there is some evidence that it may also lower your risk of colon cancer. There are side effects; the major one being an increased risk of blood clots. Blood clots can cause stroke, heart attacks, or pulmonary embolism (blood clot in the lung), all serious and potentially fatal conditions. The overall risk is very low and the good news is that the risk doesn't increase with age, *unless you are a smoker. If you smoke you should absolutely not use birth control pills.*

Along with smoking, you should not use OCPs if you have any of the following:

- Blood clotting disorder
- Migraine headaches, particularly with aura
- Cerebrovascular or coronary artery disease
- Uncontrolled hypertension
- Dyslipidemia unresponsive to therapy
- Breast or uterine cancer
- Certain liver diseases or liver cancer
- Diabetes with nerve, vascular, eye, or kidney damage
- Prolonged immobilization

You can safely use OCPs into your early 50s. One issue with using OCPs through perimenopause is figuring out when you've reached menopause. You will continue to have a period as long as you are taking OCPs. One option is to remain on the pill until age 55, when it becomes very unlikely that you are still ovulating. Your health care provider can check your hormone levels after you have been off the pill for a month; elevated levels of follicle stimulating hormone indicate menopause has been reached.

Safe Sex

A mistake older women make too often, and one that can be devastating, is assuming that older means safer when it comes to sexually transmitted diseases. One of the joys of sex after

What Nurses Know...

STI Statistics

HIV/AIDS

- *42,495 new cases of HIV/AIDS diagnosed in 2007*
  - *Females made up 26 percent of these cases*
  - *Heterosexual sexual contact was responsible for 83 percent of cases in women*
  - *44 percent of new cases were in people 40 years of age and older; 17 percent of them were in people 50 years of age and older*

Gonorrhea and syphilis are less common

- *25,468 total cases of gonorrhea in people 40 and older in 2008*

- *4,368 cases of syphilis in people 40 and older in 2008*

menopause is that it can be carefree. Carefree doesn't mean careless. You should be as careful about protection as your daughter or niece or the college kid next door.

Vaginal atrophy makes you more vulnerable to STIs that are transmitted through contact with blood such as HIV and hepatitis B. Dry, thin vaginal tissues are more prone to tear and bleed during intercourse, providing an opening for organisms to enter.

So talk to your partner about his or her sexual history and use a condom with a new male partner until you know for sure that he is disease-free. That means until he's been tested for STIs, including AIDS and hepatitis B, and you've seen a copy of the results.

Lesbian women need protection with new partners as well. Use a latex barrier for vulva contact and oral sex. If you share sex toys, use condoms or wash with hot soapy water between users.

Remember the oft repeated but very true adage when it comes to STIs—you are sleeping with everyone your partner has ever slept with. Insisting on using barriers may not seem like the most romantic move when things get heated up, but it beats the heck out of discovering you've been infected with something that will turn your life upside down or even kill you.

What Nurses Know...

Be in control of your own sex life. Carry condoms with you. Unplanned spontaneous sex is when the use of a condom is least likely to happen. Be prepared to safely take advantage of those spontaneous moments of passion.

Resources

The Alexander Foundation for Women's Health

The Web site for this nonprofit organization includes links to numerous articles on women's health, including menopause and sexuality. It also has links to Web sites of many other women's organizations.

www.afwh.org

The American Association of Sexuality Educators, Counselors and Therapists

The Web site for this professional organization includes a list of sex therapists and counselors.

www.aasect.org

North American Menopause Society

The Web site of the professional organization has a consumer section that includes information on sexual issues. There is also an Ask the Experts section with questions and answers about sexuality.

www.menopause.org

Bone Health

I was about 60 when I found out I had osteoporosis. My doctor was suspicious because I was thin and ordered a bone density test. I hadn't shrunk at all or had any outward signs. Since then, though, I've shrunk an inch and I have a small curvature of the spine. That's the worst part, the shrinking and the fear of being bent over and stooping. MARY

Osteoporosis

Osteoporosis is a major cause of disability and death in older women. Our bones are strongest when we are about 30 years of age. Until then we have a balanced bone turnover; new bone cells take over for those that are destroyed, maintaining healthy strong bone tissue. After the age of 30, though, our production of new cells doesn't quite keep up with the destruction of old cells, and our bones begin to lose density and steadily weaken.

● ●

Stat Facts

- 15 percent of women older than 50 years of age have osteoporosis
- 33 percent of women between 60 and 70 years of age have osteoporosis
- 66 percent of women older than 80 years of age have osteoporosis
- 45 percent of women older than 50 years of age have osteopenia.

The rate of bone mass loss varies among women, but by the time we reach 80 years of age most of us have lost about 30 percent of our bone mass. Brittle bones break more easily. A fall that would have left us with only a bruise in our 30s can result in a broken hip in our 70s.

A number of factors determine each woman's individual rate of bone loss. These include genetics, diet, calcium and vitamin D intake, and exercise. Loss of estrogen has a major impact on bone loss. After menopause the rate of bone loss increases dramatically. Women with early menopause, before the age of 45, have a much higher risk of osteoporosis.

Maybe you can't control things like early menopause or your genes, but you certainly can do something about the other factors. What you do now can mean the difference between disability or dancing in your later years.

Osteopenia

Osteopenia and osteoporosis both mean low bone mass density (BMD); it's just a matter of how low. Osteopenia is decreased bone density that is not as severe as osteoporosis. It is a warning sign for women that they are at risk for osteoporosis. A diagnosis of osteopenia does not automatically mean you should be on medication. In fact, current recommendations are against treating most women with osteopenia with medication. Only women at increased risk of osteoporotic fractures should be treated. You and your health care provider need to determine if you have additional risk factors for osteoporosis that indicate you would benefit from medication to enhance your bone health.

The World Health Organization has developed a risk assessment tool called FRAX for women with osteopenia. It uses your individual risk factors to calculate your risk for breaking a hip or other major bone over the next 10 years due to osteoporosis. Experts recommend treatment if the 10-year risk for a hip fracture is three percent or higher or 20 percent or higher for a major osteoporotic fracture. There are computer tools that will do the calculation. Software is being added to bone densitometry scan machines so the calculation can be done with the bone density test. Ask your health care provider about calculating your FRAX® score when you talk to him or her about osteoporosis.

FRAX® Calculation

FRAX® uses the following factors to calculate your risk of a hip or other major osteoporotic fracture in the next 10 years:

- Age
- Weight
- Height
- Previous fracture
- Parent fractured hip
- Current smoking
- Glucocorticoids
- Rheumatoid arthritis
- Secondary osteoporosis
- Alcohol three or more units per day
- Femoral neck BMD (result of bone densitometry scan).

Osteopenia may not mean you have to take medication, but it does mean you have to pay attention. You need to make sure you engage in lifestyle measures to prevent advancing to osteoporosis.

What Nurses Know...

Be prepared to talk to your health care provider about your risk of osteoporosis. Gather the following information before your visit:

- *Family history of osteoporosis. Has either of your parents fractured their hip?*

- *Keep a food diary for two weeks. This will help determine your calcium intake.*

- *Current medication list. Include supplements and herbal preparations.*

- *Time since menopause*

- *Estrogen therapy*

- *History of long-term use of prednisone or other glucocorticoids*

- *History of chemotherapy*

- *History of eating disorder*

- *Alcohol use*

- *Activity level and exercise routine*

Determining Risk

I'm from Ireland and there were no tests done there for osteoporosis when I was younger, but I think my mother had it. She was very thin and shrunk a lot in her later days. And she had been such a tall woman. I'd say she went from 5'7" to 5'3" in her lifetime.   MARY

There are a number of factors that put you at increased risk for osteoporosis and osteoporosis-related fractures. Check out the list below. If you have any of these it means you have a greater *chance* of having osteoporosis; it does *not* mean that you have it. Every woman should take measures to ensure bone health regardless of risk, but women with these risk factors need to be especially committed to preventive action.

● ●

Risk Factors for Osteoporosis

The presence of any of the following indicate an increased risk of osteoporosis:

- History of a fracture from an injury that ordinarily should not cause a fracture
- Family history of osteoporosis
- Early menopause
- White or Asian race
- Lack of weight-bearing exercise
- Too much intense exercise, especially endurance exercises like marathon running
- Low body weight
- Low calcium intake in diet
- Long periods of bed rest during an illness or injury
- Alcoholism
- Eating disorders
- Kidney or liver disease
- Smoking
- Frailty
- Long-term use of prednisone
- Malabsorption illnesses such as Crohn's or sprue disease

MEASURING BONE MINERAL DENSITY

You can get a more accurate assessment of your risks with a bone density scan. Bone densitometry tests measure your BMD. The most common bone densitometry test used is a dual emission X-ray absorptiometry (DEXA or DXA) scan of your spine and hips. The test is painless and usually takes about 10 minutes to perform. X-ray exposure is minimal.

• •

Who Needs Bone Densitometry Testing?

Not every postmenopausal woman needs bone densitometry testing. According to recommendations from the North American Menopause Society (NAMS) and the National Osteoporosis Foundation, bone densitometry should be done in the following women:

- All postmenopausal women who have had a fracture
- All women with medical causes of bone loss such as those who have had chemotherapy or used glucocorticoids long term
- All women age 65 or older
- Women younger than age 65 who have one or more risk factors

The DEXA scan reports your density as a *Z*-score or a *T*-score. If you are under the age of 50 and premenopausal your BMD will be reported with a *Z*-score. The *Z*-score compares the difference between your bone density and the average *Z*-score for women of your age and ethnicity. If you are over 50 and postmenopausal your BMD will be reported as a *T*-score. The *T*-score is the difference between your score and the average score for a healthy 30-year-old woman. Race and ethnicity are not considered in the calculation of a *T*-score.

There is another way to diagnose osteoporosis, one you want to avoid—falling and sustaining a fracture due to brittle bones. Unfortunately, this is the way many women find out they have osteoporosis. There are no symptoms to warn you that your bones are getting brittle.

There are a number of actions you can take to keep your bones healthy and prevent fractures. Now is the time to get your bones strong for the rest of your life. There are two ways to do that. The first and best way is through lifestyle measures. The second option, though only appropriate in a select group of women, is with medications that enhance bone density.

I've always been active but now I walk more. I need to keep active, keep walking. I take calcium and a nose spray called

Miacalcin. As a result of all this my bones have thickened. At my last appointment, on the bone density test, they saw that it had improved significantly. So I'll continue doing what I'm doing and get tested every two years. MARY

Lifestyle Measures for Bone Health

There are two lifestyle measures that are essential in maintaining bone health. Your diet, especially calcium and vitamin D, is the first. The other is weight-bearing exercise.

Also, if you're a smoker, quit. Along with all of the other ill effects of smoking, add bone loss. If you are a smoker there really is no other one thing you can do that will have as great a positive impact on your health. Talk to your health care provider about help with quitting. There are options: support groups, hypnosis, acupuncture, and medication have helped many people finally quit the habit. If you have tried and failed, don't give up on it. Few people quit for good on the first try.

Heavy alcohol use is a risk factor for osteoporosis, as well. If you drink more than two glasses a day you are increasing your risk. For optimal health, limit your alcohol to no more than one of the following a day: four ounces of wine, 12 ounces of beer, or one ounce of liquor.

DIET

The most important thing you can do for bone health is to ensure that you get enough calcium and vitamin D. Calcium is the primary mineral responsible for bone strength. The chief food source is dairy products. Vitamin D is needed for your body to absorb the calcium it takes in. Vitamin D is found in a few foods, but it is primarily produced through natural sunlight exposure.

Calcium Sufficient calcium is essential for healthy bones. Postmenopausal women who get enough calcium have less risk of osteoporosis and fractures. As we get older our bodies get less efficient in using the calcium we take in. The loss of estrogen further reduces our bones' ability to absorb the calcium they need.

Along with strong bones, calcium has a few added bonuses. There is evidence that suggests it helps protect against colon cancer and also may help lower blood pressure. And it may even help fight those extra pounds that want to creep on after menopause. Studies show that the less calcium a person has in their diet, the higher the risk of obesity.

After menopause, the recommended calcium intake varies. If you are younger than 65 and using estrogen you should get 1,000 milligrams per day. If you are not using estrogen or are older than 65 years of age, then you need 1,500 milligrams per day. Getting enough calcium is not difficult, yet few women do. Two or three cups of milk or another dairy product are all it takes to meet the daily requirement.

There are no tests to check your calcium level. Keep a food diary for a couple of weeks and check it against the list of foods that contain calcium. There are no known benefits to taking more calcium than the recommended daily requirement. In fact, it can increase your risk of gastrointestinal (GI) distress and kidney stones.

Most of us don't have to worry about calcium causing kidney stones, unless we take more than the recommended requirement. There is some evidence that maintaining the optimal level of calcium may actually help prevent kidney stones. Calcium binds to the primary component of stones, oxalic acid, in your intestines. If you or a family member has a history of kidney stones avoid foods that are high in oxalic acid, spinach is among the highest, and drink plenty of water while on calcium supplements.

Ideally, your calcium supply should come from food. The best dietary source of calcium is dairy products. They are not only high in calcium, but also the calcium is better absorbed than that which is in other food. It is not known how well our bodies absorb the calcium we get from calcium-fortified foods.

If you are a strict vegetarian, lactose-intolerant, or have a poor diet, then you probably do not get enough calcium in your diet. You should take calcium supplements.

Dietary Sources of Calcium

- Dairy products

  - Milk
  - Cheese
  - Yogurt

- Vegetables

  - Broccoli
  - Collards
  - Soybeans
  - Turnip greens
  - Kidney beans
  - Refried beans
  - Tofu

- Almonds
- Salmon, canned with bones
- Sardines, in oil with bones

There are many types of calcium supplements. The two most common are calcium carbonate and calcium citrate. One is not necessarily better than the other. When reading the label of any calcium supplement, you want to pay attention to the level of *elemental calcium* in the product. This is the amount that is considered in the recommended daily level. Each type of calcium contains a different level of "elemental calcium."

What Nurses Know...

If you are taking iron supplements, do not take them with calcium supplements. Calcium lowers the rate of iron absorption.

To maximize absorption you should always take calcium supplements with food and in divided doses. Do not take more than 500 milligrams of calcium at a time. More of the calcium will be absorbed and it is less likely to upset your stomach.

GI upset is the most common complaint women have about taking calcium supplements. If you have stomach upset even when you take a calcium supplement with food, try dividing the dose or switching to a different form. There are all kinds of options; tablets, chocolate and caramel-flavored chews, dissolvable tablets, and liquids. Many women take chewable calcium carbonate antacid tablets as their calcium supplement.

Vitamin D   Recent research has highlighted the importance of vitamin D in maintaining our health. Not only do we need vitamin D in order for our bodies to use calcium, it also appears to play a role in preventing cancer, heart disease, mental illness, lung disease, and Type I diabetes.

Vitamin D is essential in maintaining strong bones and preventing fractures. If you do not have enough vitamin D, your body only absorbs about 10 to 15 percent of the calcium you take in. Vitamin D also prevents fractures through its effect on muscle strength. When your muscles are weak you are more prone to falls, which all too often result in fractures if you have osteoporosis.

Vitamin D deficiency can also cause another bone condition, called osteomalacia. Instead of brittle bones associated with osteoporosis, in osteomalacia your bones soften. And whereas

What Nurses Know...

If you see the prefix osteo, *then the word has something to do with your bones.*

osteoporosis is painless, osteomalacia often causes throbbing and aching bone pain.

Unlike calcium, vitamin D levels can be checked with a blood test. Tests measure the level of 25-hydroxyvitamin D in your blood. Current recommendations state that it should be at least 30 nanograms per milliliter. However, newer information indicates this is not enough, and most experts now believe we need to aim for higher levels, as high as 75 nanograms per milliliter.

Though thinking about recommended dietary intake of vitamin D has changed, advice from the health care community has not kept up. One reason may be concerns about toxicity. Vitamin D is a fat-soluble vitamin, so excess amounts build up in your system. This differs from water-soluble vitamins, such as vitamin C, where your body uses what it needs and gets rid of the rest in your urine. However, research shows that the safety margin for vitamin D is much higher than previously thought, as much as 10 times higher.

We get vitamin D from sunlight, vitamin-D-enriched foods, and supplements. Sunlight is the biggest source of vitamin D. The amount of sun exposure you need depends on the time of year, where you live, and your skin color. However, unless you live near the equator, it's unlikely you get enough for adequate vitamin D production. And if you live in the northeast it is virtually impossible during winter months. Other times of the year, if you are fair-skinned you can produce enough vitamin D with about 10 minutes of sun exposure in the middle of the day a few days a week. If you have dark skin you need 5 to 10 times that much. You also need much more exposure if you use sunscreen with a sun protection factor (SPF) of eight or more, which can reduce vitamin D production by 95 percent. All of these exposure times are based on wearing clothes that expose your legs and arms. Since few of us are wandering around in shorts and a tank top every day, it is very unlikely that we are getting enough sun exposure for adequate vitamin D production.

There are few dietary sources of vitamin D outside of fortified foods. Unless you're eating oily fish every day you won't be able to get

What Nurses Know...

Be careful taking omega-3 fatty acid supplements. You should avoid those made with fish oil; they contain unknown levels of vitamin A. It has been found that too much vitamin A can be bad for your bones. Flaxseed oil is a better source of omega-3 fatty acid.

enough vitamin D from diet alone. Foods with the highest levels of vitamin D are salmon, mackerel, and tuna. The other dietary source of vitamin D is fortified foods, but none of these reach the level of vitamin D found in oily fish. When reading food labels remember that until the Food and Drug Administration (FDA) changes their recommendations, the percentage of daily value is based on levels that are less than what experts currently recommend.

It is estimated that over 50 percent of postmenopausal women are deficient in vitamin D.

Talk to your health care provider about getting a blood test to check your vitamin D level. The level of supplementation should be based on those results. Many women will need to take higher doses for a few months to get their level up before continuing with a maintenance dose.

Once you know your vitamin D level, talk to your health care provider about the amount of supplementation, if any, you should

Alert

DO NOT take mega doses of vitamin D on your own! Though the safety margin is higher than previously thought, there is still a risk of toxicity and certain chronic illnesses can make you more sensitive to vitamin D.

be taking. Current recommendations of 400 to 600 International Units a day just aren't enough to provide your body with what is now considered the optimum level of vitamin D. You will probably need about 1,000 International Units. There are different types of vitamin D supplements. The most effective is vitamin D3 (cholecalciferol). You need almost three times as much vitamin D2 to equal what your body gets from vitamin D3 supplements.

We now know that getting enough vitamin D is critical for our overall health. Bone health is just the beginning; it affects almost every system of our bodies. Do not neglect this important aspect of your health. Especially when it's so easy to get it right!

WEIGHT-BEARING EXERCISE

Weight-bearing exercise is essential for maintaining bone health. Research shows that exercise, particularly weight-bearing exercise, increases bone mass in the spine and hips of women with postmenopausal osteoporosis. These are the two areas that women with osteoporosis have the most problems with.

• •

Running: Getting Started

Running is great weight-bearing exercise for bone health. Almost anyone can run, anywhere. You don't need a gym membership or special equipment. All it costs is the price of a good pair of running shoes. *The key is to start slow and build up gradually.* Here are a few tips to get started.

Alternate running and walking. Start off alternating walking 10 minutes and running one or two minutes. Each week gradually increase the time spent running and decrease the time spent walking until you are running the entire distance. Then start increasing the total distance.

Set a finish line marker for yourself and every few days run another 10 feet past it.

Set a goal that you are working toward. Enter a short-distance race six months from your starting date and work toward that.

Get yourself a running partner.

Run at the same time each day. Treat it like any other important appointment.

Gradually work up to running at a pace that makes talking difficult but not impossible.

Listen to your body. DO NOT try to run through pain.

Brisk walking is great exercise for overall fitness and weight control. It also helps maintain bone mass. Walking for one hour, four times a week has been shown to decrease bone loss. To increase bone mass though, you need activities that are high impact such as running and jump-roping. It appears that the higher the impact, the more your bones respond positively. Short bursts of repeated activity that is site-specific, that "load" on certain bones, is best. Don't expect miracles; even high-impact exercise will result in only about a two percent increase in bone mass.

You should always talk to your health care provider before starting any exercise program, and this is no exception. If you have any risk factors for osteoporosis and haven't had a bone density test done, it is a good idea to get one before you decide to start jumping around in an aerobics class. If you already have significant osteoporosis, intense high-impact exercise can put you at risk for a fracture.

Meanwhile, get up out of your chair! Start moving. Though walking won't *increase* your bone mass it will help *maintain* what you have. It will also help with muscle strength and balance, both key in preventing falls and subsequent fractures. And you will reap the added benefits of improved cardiovascular health and stress relief.

All the high-impact exercise in the world won't help you, though, if you aren't getting enough calcium. Exercise helps your bones absorb and hold onto calcium. Neither is very effective without the other.

Medications

Medications are an appropriate option for a select group of women. The available medications include estrogen, bisphosphonates, selective estrogen receptor modulators (SERMs), and calcitonin.

ESTROGEN
Estrogen is very effective in maintaining bone density. Prevention of osteoporosis is the only indication that has FDA approval for *long-term* use of estrogen. Estrogen will prevent bone loss and

slow down further loss in women who already have osteoporosis. Check out Chapters 7 and 8 for in-depth information about estrogen and estrogen use.

BISPHOSPHONATES

Bisphosphonates are drugs that slow down the activity of osteoclasts, the cells that break down bone. They are effective in slowing or stopping the loss of bone density. There are a number of bisphosphonates used in the United States for the treatment of osteoporosis: alendronate (Fosamax), ibandronate (Boniva), risedronate (Actonel), and zoledronic (Reclast). Ibandronate and zoledronic come in an intravenous form for women who can't tolerate oral forms.

Bisphosphonates come in different strengths and dosing schedules, so you can choose a form that you take daily, once or twice a week, monthly, once every three months, or once a year. Bisphosphonates should only be used in women who have adequate calcium and good kidney function. Make sure you have blood work to check your kidney function before starting on bisphosphonates. You should also not take bisphosphonates if you have bad heartburn or problems with your esophagus. The most common problems women have with the medication are heartburn and gastritis. Unfortunately, bisphosphonates have to be taken only with water on an empty stomach to be effective, making it difficult to manage these side effects. A few women on a high dose of bisphosphonates will experience a mild flu-like illness when they take their first dose; it passes without any lasting effects.

However, there have been reports of some women experiencing more serious side effects, including severe bone, joint, and muscle pain, osteonecrosis of the jaw, and unusual femur fractures. As with any medication it is very important to weigh the risk versus benefit before starting treatment with bisphosphonates. Bisphosphonates can cause serious problems, but so can osteoporosis. You and your health care provider must decide your individual risk versus benefit profile before making a decision about bisphosphonate use.

Severe Bone, Joint, and Muscle Pain   Severe and sometimes incapacitating bone, joint, and muscle pain has been reported in women taking bisphosphonates, usually those older than 65 years. Usually the pain resolves once they stop taking the medication, but sometimes it can take awhile, and in some cases it never goes completely away. If you have new onset or worsening of preexisting bone, joint, or muscle pain anytime after starting bisphosphonates, stop taking the medication and report it to your health care provider right away. This can develop right away or even months or years after starting the medicine.

Osteonecrosis of the Jaw   There are reports of cases of osteonecrosis of the jaw in people taking bisphosphonates. Osteonecrosis of the jaw is a rare disorder where tissue in the jaw dies, exposing bone. The area does not heal or may heal only after a long period of time. Pain and infection may occur. Almost 95 percent of the cases have been in patients on chemotherapy who are taking bisphosphonates to treat cancer that has spread to the bone. However, it does happen in people taking bisphosphonates for osteoporosis. It usually happens in people who have dental disease or following a dental procedure. This is a rare occurrence overall. If you are taking bisphosphonates talk to your health care provider about your personal risks before deciding to stop the medication. Make sure you get regular dental care to maintain good dental health.

Atypical Femur Fractures   There have also been reports of unusual (atypical) fractures of the femur (thigh bone) just below the hip in women taking bisphosphonates. It happens so infrequently, though, that it's been difficult to tell if the fractures are related to the medication or not. In March 2010 the FDA released an announcement stating that currently there are no data that show a "clear connection" between bisphosphonates and this particular type of fracture, but research is continuing.

These last two problems have raised concerns about the effects of long-term bisphosphonate use. Experts are questioning if they cause too much suppression of bone turnover with

Who Should Receive Medication to Treat Osteoporosis?

According to recommendations from NAMS, treatment with medication to increase bone density should be limited to the following women:

● All postmenopausal women with bone density scan *T*-scores less than −2.5
● Postmenopausal women with bone density scan *T*-scores from −2.0 to −2.5 and one or more risk factors
● All postmenopausal women with a history of a vertebral or hip fracture.

long-term use, leading to weaker bones over time. The FDA and researchers are continuing to explore this and other questions about the safe and effective use of bisphosphonates.

SELECTIVE ESTROGEN RECEPTOR MODULATORS

Selective estrogen receptor modulators (SERMs) are medications that act just like estrogen on some tissues of the body, while also acting to block the effects of estrogen on other tissues. They were first used in the treatment of breast cancer because they block estrogen from acting on breast tissue. They attach to estrogen receptors in breast tissue so estrogen can't. Remember from Chapter 2, estrogen is a hormone that has no activity of its own; it has to attach to its target cell to carry out its purpose. You may have heard of tamoxifen; it is the oldest, most often prescribed SERM for the treatment of breast cancer. At the present time there is only one SERM approved for the treatment of osteoporosis in the United States, raloxifene (Evista).

SERMs are used to treat osteoporosis because they stimulate estrogen receptors in bone tissue. (Hence the term *selective*, because they act *selectively* on different tissues.) The most common side effects of SERMs are hot flashes (not welcome news for menopausal women) and leg cramps. SERMs do not increase the risk for breast cancer (in fact, they appear to lower your risk of invasive breast cancer) and endometrial cancer like estrogen does, but they do increase the risk of blood clots in the veins. You should not take SERMs if you have ever had a blood clot or if you have risk factors for stroke.

CALCITONIN

Calcitonin is a hormone produced by the thyroid gland that acts to slow down the release of calcium from bones. It is available as a medication, calcitonin salmon, that is made from calcitonin extracted from salmon. It is used for the treatment of osteoporosis of the spine, especially for vertebral fractures, in women who are at least five years past menopause. It has no effect on hip or other nonvertebral fractures and should not be used for these purposes. It is effective in relieving pain after a compression fracture of the vertebra (see below for more information on this condition) in women with osteoporosis.

Calcitonin salmon is available as a nasal spray or a subcutaneous injection (injection just under the skin with a very small needle). It is not as effective as other medications for osteoporosis and is usually not prescribed, other than for osteoporosis of the spine, unless you are unable to tolerate other medications.

Osteoporotic Fractures

The biggest threats of osteoporosis are hip and vertebral fractures. Hip fractures are especially concerning. They cause serious health

• •

Stat Facts

- 90 percent of hip and spine fractures in older women are a result of osteoporosis
- Osteoporosis causes 1.5 million fractures a year in the United States
- 40 percent of women over 50 years of age will have a fracture as a result of osteoporosis
- Over 90 percent of hip fractures are caused by falling
- There is a 25 percent increased death rate in the year following a hip fracture
- About one in five people who fracture their hip dies within a year of the injury
- One in four people who lived on their own before a hip fracture spend at least a year in a nursing home after their injury
- Hip fractures result in long-term disability in 50 percent of survivors.

problems for older women and can lead to prolonged disability and even early death. Vertebral fractures can cause significant chronic back pain and reduce your ability to do everyday activities.

HIP FRACTURES

Hip fractures are probably the most dreaded outcome of osteoporosis. As evident by the statistics above, disability and death too often follow them. Most hip fractures occur in women in their early 80s, but prevention should start long before then. Taking the measures needed for optimal bone strength is one part of a triangle of prevention. Second is staying physically fit and maintaining balance and flexibility to prevent injuries that can cause broken bones. And third is taking precautions to make sure your environment is safe.

What Nurses Know . . .

Preventing falls is the key to preventing fractures. *Take the following steps to lower your risk of falls:*

- *Exercise regularly to maintain strength and coordination*

- *Do yoga to increase flexibility and balance*

- *Avoid sedatives and other medications, like antihistamines, that can cause dizziness*

- *Have annual eye examinations*

- *Make sure your surroundings are well lit*

- *Keep halls and entryways clear of obstacles*

- *Avoid throw rugs or use double-sided tape or nonslip pads to keep rugs in place*

- *Do not leave items on the floor*

- *Keep stairways clear and in good repair*

- *Keep wires and cords next to the wall, not stretched across the floor*

- *Use a nonslip mat in the tub and shower*

- *Don't try to overreach for items*

- *Always use a step-stool or ladder, not a chair or other makeshift elevation*

VERTEBRAL FRACTURES

Hip fractures may be the most dreaded of outcomes, but vertebral fractures are the most common. And they too can have significant effects on your quality of life.

Osteoporotic vertebral fractures are compression fractures. The vertebra collapse onto themselves, flattening out. Women with compression fractures become shorter. Some women end up bent over, what used to be known as a dowager's hump (the medical term for this is kyphosis). Recent research shows that women who have lost an inch and a half of height are highly likely to have one or more vertebral fractures. Most of us can expect to become shorter as we get older, usually by about one to three inches, but it should not be more than half an inch about every 10 years, at least till age 70, when the rate may pick up. Until then any loss greater than half an inch warrants further investigation.

Pain with vertebral compression fractures varies among women. When the fracture occurs, you may feel a sudden sharp pain or you may feel nothing. You may not know what is causing that persistent pain in your back, or put it off to too much hard work or a new exercise routine. For some women the pain becomes chronic and severe while others have little or no pain. It is important to find out if you have suffered a compression fracture. Not only do you need appropriate treatment for the injury,

What Nurses Know...

Most of us do not accurately report our height. You should have a height measurement done each year. Make sure when you visit your health care provider that they do a height measurement, not just ask you what your height is.

but without follow-up you are also at increased risk for further fractures and decreased physical functioning.

Treatment for a vertebral compression fracture is directed at relieving pain and maintaining function. Nonsteroidal anti-inflammatory drugs (NSAIDs) are effective for mild-to-moderate pain. Severe pain may need an opioid pain killer. As noted earlier, calcitonin salmon is used for pain relief as well. Bed rest is not the best thing for back pain. If needed, it should be for the shortest time possible, preferably a day or two at most. Staying active is best, just no vigorous activity.

Treatment should also include prevention of further fractures. If you have not had a bone densitometry or are not being treated for osteoporosis already, you need to talk to your health care provider about doing so.

Prevention is really the key when it comes to osteoporosis. Developing the lifestyle habits that enhance bone health should begin as early as possible, ideally in childhood. But it is never too late.

Resources

International Osteoporosis Foundation
The Web site for this international organization offers information about osteoporosis and a short online test to find out your risk status. Click on the link for Patients and Public. www.iofbonehealth.org/

National Osteoporosis Foundation

The Web site for this nonprofit organization dedicated to bone health has information on osteoporosis, support groups for people with osteoporosis, and information on finding a health care provider who is an expert in osteoporosis.

www.nof.org/

Office of Dietary Supplements

This National Institutes of Health (NIH) Web site offers extensive information on dietary supplement use. Click on the Health Information link on the home page. On the top right there is a section on Specific Supplements where you will find fact sheets for calcium and vitamin D.

http://dietary-supplements.info.nih.gov

Osteoporosis and Related Bone Diseases National Resource Center

This NIH Web site has information on bone health and osteoporosis, and links to numerous resources.

www.osteo.org/

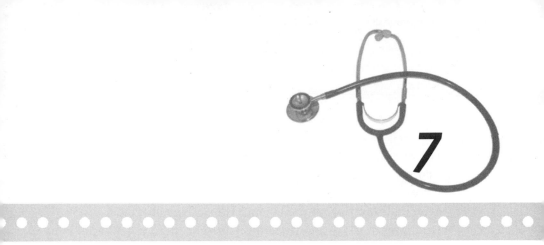

Hormone Therapy: What We Know Now and What It Means for You

Estrogen, it's magic. I dread the day I have to stop it.   FRAN

I don't want to use estrogen. Menopause is a natural part of life. I want to let nature take its course.   SUE

I'd use estrogen in a minute if I didn't have bad migraines. I've tried all those other things people tell you to try and nothing's worked for me.   KRISTINE

If hormone replacement therapy is not an option for symptoms, then what is? My gynecologist suggested soy phytoestrogen, which made me have a raging PMS attack.   JOYCE

Estrogen therapy (ET) has a long and uneven history: from a cure-all for the "deficiency disease" of menopause to a cancer-causing pariah. As with most things, the truth lies somewhere in between.

"Every woman has to decide for herself." If you have talked to your health care provider recently about taking estrogen for menopausal symptoms, you have probably heard this. It is common practice for health care providers to expect women to make their own decision about ET after being given all the latest information. Making sense of all the latest facts and figures, and figuring out exactly what it all means for you, is not easy.

Adding to the difficulty is the fact that there is still a lot of debate going on in the scientific community about the safety and effectiveness of ET. You will find a few people at either extreme of the debate. Some advise against any use of estrogen and others think the concerns have been blown way out of proportion. But most experts now believe there is a place for ET, with careful consideration given to each individual woman's situation.

The Other Hormones—Testosterone and DHEA

Estrogen is not the only hormone used to treat distressing aspects of menopause; there are also testosterone and dehydroepiandrosterone (DHEA). Both of these are shrouded in uncertainty and controversy, as well.

Testosterone has received a lot of attention lately, especially in the treatment of sexual problems during the menopausal transition and after menopause. You will also see it touted as a cure for low energy, hot flashes, depression, and osteoporosis. There is still little good information available about its effectiveness and safety. At the present time it is only recommended for treatment of problems with sexual desire and response in menopausal women, and only when used in combination with estrogen. (See Chapter 5 for a full discussion of testosterone and sexuality.) There is not enough evidence to support using it for any other purpose.

There is even less known about DHEA, a newer hormonal supplement gaining attention. There is very little good research on the effectiveness and safety of DHEA use in postmenopausal women. Some evidence is starting to accumulate that indicates it may help prevent osteoporosis, but questions remain. Other than that, there is little to support claims that it improves well-being or sexual function. There are also mixed results from studies looking at its effect on the risk of heart disease, breast cancer, and the uterus. At this time the use of DHEA in postmenopausal women is not recommended. Too little is known about its effectiveness or potential side effects.

There are all kinds of Web sites promoting testosterone and DHEA treatment for a variety of purposes: to delay aging, to enhance your well-being, or to increase your libido. Some Web sites present themselves as informational, but be careful. Most are advertisements in disguise and their main purpose is to sell you their product. The information they provide is biased to increase sales.

What We're Talking About When We Talk About Hormone Therapy

Hormone therapy (HT) is often referred to as hormone replacement therapy in the media, in biomedical literature, and by health care providers. This is inaccurate and does not conform to current Food and Drug Administration (FDA) regulations. Estrogen supplements are just that—supplements. They do not "replace" anywhere near the amount of estrogen that was produced by the ovaries premenopause, nor do combinations of estrogen and a progestogen "replace" the complex hormonal arrangement maintained by the body during the reproductive years. The official terminology, which will be used throughout this book, is as follows:

- *ET* for estrogen therapy (not supplementation)
- *EPT for combined estrogen-plus-progestogen therapy*
- *HT* for either ET or EPT

Hormone Therapy—The Basics

This section will give a general review of HT and options for treatment. For a full discussion of the risks versus benefits, see the section on the Women's Health Initiative (WHI) study below.

• •

A Brief History of HT: Drugs in Search of a Disease

It all started with men in ancient civilizations eating the penis and testicles of animals as a cure for impotence. Another early form of hormonal treatments was urine drinking, practiced by ancient yogis. Later, Chinese chemists distilled large volumes of urine in preparation for use in a number of conditions, including impotence.

The modern day story of estrogen began in 1923, when an "ovarian hormone" was isolated for the first time. This hormone, named estrogen, came to be seen as the source of femininity, and menopause increasingly came to be seen as a disease of estrogen deficiency, often blamed for many age-related problems, as well. The use of estrogen was not widespread yet, however, because there just wasn't enough of it to go around. In 1925 it was found that estrogen could be extracted from the urine of pregnant women, but this method yielded only a limited supply. That changed in 1943, when estrogen was first extracted from the urine of pregnant mares, allowing for large quantities to be produced. Soon Premarin entered the market. Now there was a supply—time to create a demand.

That happened in the 1960s with the publication of the book, *Feminine Forever* by Dr. Robert Wilson, a New York gynecologist. Dr. Wilson also published a number of articles in medical journals with titles like "The Obsolete Menopause" and "The Fate of the Nontreated Postmenopausal Woman: A Plea for the Maintenance of Adequate Estrogen From Puberty to the Grave," describing postmenopausal women as "castrates" and calling for medical treatment of women "suffering from estrogen deficiency." Drug companies happily backed him as he traveled the country promoting estrogen as an antiaging drug, one that would save women from the "living decay" of menopause; not only to save women from themselves but also to save society from "the untold misery of alcoholism, drug addiction, divorce, and broken homes caused by these unstable, estrogen-starved women."

Not all physicians agreed with the concept that menopause was a medical condition or that estrogen was the answer. In fact, many argued for restraint in the use of estrogen and some for avoidance of it altogether. Most experts agreed that more research was needed before any conclusions could be made about the safety or usefulness of ET in menopausal women.

Also, the publication of *Feminine Forever* happened in the context of the 60s and the drug culture, not just the illegal use of so-called psychedelics and other street drugs. Prescriptions for all drugs doubled during this time. People came to expect a magic pill for everything that ailed them. Estrogen filled that expectation almost perfectly for the "conditions" of menopause and aging.

Estrogen sales skyrocketed. By 1975, Premarin was the second most widely prescribed drug on the market.

Then the first hints surfaced that all was not well in the "feminine forever" world. Studies indicated that taking estrogen increased the risk of cancer of the endometrium (the uterine lining). Sales fell through the late 1970s and into the early 1980s until drug manufacturers found that adding progesterone to estrogen products solved that problem. Once again women started taking estrogen products as a matter of routine, and not just for hot flashes or other difficult aspects of menopause—it was also taken as an antiaging medication, touted to hold off everything from wrinkles to Alzheimer's. (A gynecologist I worked with from the 1990s through 2002 used to prescribe it as a matter of course to all his female patients as soon as they hit 46 years of age to "prevent" menopause.) Bolstered by reports that HT protected against heart disease, osteoporosis and cancer, the estrogen business was back on track and, with the baby boomer generation now in their 40s and 50s, getting bigger all the time. By 2000, Premarin was again the second most frequently prescribed medication in the United States. Its sales brought in over one billion dollars.

And then the bomb dropped. In the spring of 2002 the National Institutes of Health (NIH) stopped a large clinical trial, the estrogen and progestin component of the WHI study. The trial was studying the effect of menopausal HT on heart disease; osteoporosis; dementia; blood clots; and breast, uterine, endometrial, and colon cancers. It was stopped because results showed an increased risk of breast cancer, heart attack, stroke, and blood clots in women taking estrogen or estrogen-plus-progestin over women taking a placebo. (A follow-up study of the women in the WHI study is due to finish in 2010.) Many women stopped taking HT or decided not to start. A study of over 200,000 women in Britain found the rate of women using HT dropped from 29 percent in 2001 to 10 percent in 2005. A sharp drop in the number of new cases of breast cancer in 2003 was thought to be primarily caused by the decreased number of women using HT.

The history of HT is still being written. Questions abound and research continues on menopausal HT, looking at things like different types of estrogen and progesterone, or the timing and duration of therapy. It is partly driven by the pharmaceutical companies' quest for profits, but also by the fact that for some women the benefits of HT do outweigh the risks. The best news is that menopause is no longer seen as the end of femininity and estrogen is no longer viewed as the magical cure for this "deficiency disease." But HT's ideal role in menopause is still to be determined.

To read what the current recommendations are for ET, see the section on Latest Recommendations. For specifics about taking hormones, see Chapter 8.

HT is the use of estrogen or estrogen-plus-progestogen to relieve symptoms associated with menopause or to prevent unwelcome consequences. It may be used for women who have naturally occurring menopause or those with induced menopause, such as after surgery or chemotherapy.

In the United States, HT is only approved for treatment of vaginal atrophy, short-term treatment of moderate to severe hot flashes, and long-term treatment of osteoporosis. Vaginal atrophy is usually treated with vaginal estrogen, which is discussed in Chapter 5.

Hormones your body makes on its own are endogenous hormones. Endogenous means the substance is made *inside* the body by the body itself. Hormone supplements are exogenous hormones, meaning that they come from *outside* of the body.

Estrogen products contain different types of exogenous estrogen. Each type copies the structure and action of either endogenous estradiol or endogenous estrone. Conjugated estrogens like Premarin contain a combination of estrogen sources. There are slight differences in the effects of different types of estrogen; your health care provider will consider which is best for you when they prescribe an estrogen or estrogen-plus-progestogen product.

There are different types of exogenous progestogen used in estrogen-plus-progestogen products. There is also some variation in the effects of different progestogen products, especially in their action on the uterine lining and withdrawal bleeding. Some of the differences are related to how strong the progestogen is, but there may be other factors involved as well. Your health care provider will take these into consideration when choosing the appropriate estrogen-plus-progestogen product for you.

Estrogen-plus-progestogen is prescribed for women who still have a uterus. Taking oral estrogen alone for five years triples your risk of developing endometrial cancer (cancer of the uterine lining). However, vaginal estrogen and very-low-dose skin patches can be used alone if you still have your uterus.

Women who have undergone a hysterectomy and don't need to worry about endometrial cancer are prescribed estrogen alone. Estrogen taken without a progestogen is also called unopposed estrogen.

The Women's Health Initiative

The WHI was a group of studies conducted by the National Heart, Lung, and Blood Institute and the NIH beginning in 1991. The overall purpose of the initiative was to address the major health problems women encounter after menopause: heart disease, fractures, and breast and colon cancers. Different arms of the study looked at postmenopausal HT, diet, and the use of calcium and vitamin D supplements. It was a huge study, including over 161,000 women for a total of 15 years.

There were two separate studies looking at postmenopausal HT: the estrogen-plus-progestin study and the estrogen-alone study. Both studies were stopped early because early findings showed increased health risks to women receiving the hormones.

Let's take a look at each study separately and then talk about what the overall results mean for women.

What Nurses Know . . .

Understanding Research Studies

The WHI used three different types of research: observational studies, clinical trials, and community prevention studies. Observational studies "observe" events without doing anything to affect them. Community prevention studies look at the effectiveness of health prevention actions and programs. Clinical trials study the effect of treatments and other interventions given to study participants.

The research on postmenopausal HT were randomized, controlled, double-blinded clinical trials. *These are the most* reliable types of studies; they are considered the "gold standard" of research. What exactly is a randomized, controlled, double-blinded clinical trial? It's easier to understand once you know what each term means.

Randomized: *Every participant in the study has an equal chance of being put in either the group receiving the treatment or the group not receiving the treatment. So, women were randomly assigned to be in either the group taking estrogen or estrogen-plus-progestin, or in the group taking a placebo.*

Controlled: *The researchers try to "control" for factors that may affect the results of the study. One way they do this is to have the groups be very similar to each other for factors that could affect the results. Suppose the group taking estrogen had an average age of 67 and the group taking the placebo had an average age of 83. That would affect the rates of heart disease and stroke, conditions that increase as we age. By making sure that both groups have the same average age, the researchers can "control" for effects of age. Depending on what is being studied, the researchers may have to control for many different factors. Some of the more common factors include health status, race/ethnicity, educational level, and economic status.*

Double-blinded: *Neither the researcher nor the participant knows if they are taking the real treatment or are taking a placebo. This ensures that the researchers treat the women in both groups the same way and no one can do anything, purposefully or unconsciously, that may increase or decrease the effects of the treatment. For instance, if a health care provider knows their patient is taking the real treatment they may spend more time talking about side effects or monitor them more closely than a provider who knows their patient is taking a placebo and isn't concerned about harmful effects.*

ESTROGEN-PLUS-PROGESTIN STUDY

The estrogen-plus-progestin study was designed to look primarily at the effect of postmenopausal EPT on the risk of heart disease, hip fractures, and invasive breast cancer. Most of the earlier research comprised observational studies and the results were not reliable. The WHI study was also going to look at the risk of other types of cancer, stroke, and blood clots and the overall risk of death.

There were over 16,000 women from 50 to 79 years of age enrolled in the study. The group was divided almost equally between women who took an estrogen-plus-progestin tablet (Prempro) and those who took an identical-looking placebo tablet. Remember, this was a double-blinded study so neither the woman, her health care provider, or the person dispensing the tablets knew which they were taking.

All of the women were closely monitored. Follow-up phone calls, office visits, and tests were the same for both groups. The women had electrocardiograms done every three years and yearly mammograms and clinical breast examinations. About nine percent of the women had cholesterol tests done, as well.

In July 2002, after a little over five years, the NIH decided to stop the study. When the researchers looked at the information collected up to that point, it became apparent that the risks outweighed the benefits. There was a 29 percent increased risk of heart attacks and a 41 percent increase in strokes in women taking the estrogen-plus-progestin compared with those taking the placebo. The increased risk was the same for all women, regardless of whether or not she had other risk factors, like high blood pressure. Women in the estrogen-plus-progestin group also had twice the risk of having venous thrombosis, a blood clot in the veins of the legs or lungs.

Cardiovascular disease wasn't the only problem. There was a 26 percent increase in invasive breast cancer in women taking the estrogen-plus-progestin. It didn't matter if a woman had other risk factors for breast cancer. The only women who had a higher risk were those who had used postmenopausal HT before the study; in other words, those who had more exposure to estrogen. No differences in rates of endometrial cancer or lung cancer were found between the groups.

There were some benefits found, as well. Women who were taking estrogen-plus-progestin were 37 percent less likely to develop colorectal cancer. They also had a decreased risk of fractures. In the group taking estrogen-plus-progestin, there were 33 percent less hip and vertebral fractures and 24 percent less fractures overall.

After ending the study, researchers continued to examine the data and closely monitored the women involved. In 2003 they reported findings regarding dementia and quality of life that further reinforced the conclusion that risks outweighed benefits with estrogen-plus-progestin therapy. Estrogen-plus-progestin was found to double the risk of dementia, including Alzheimer's disease, in women over 65 years of age. There was no real improvement in measures of quality of life other than a very small improvement in bodily pain, sleep, and physical functioning (less than 1 point on a 100-point scale).

ESTROGEN-ALONE STUDY

The estrogen-alone study was designed to look at claims that ET decreased the risk of heart disease and increased the risk of breast cancer. Again, most of the previous research comprised observational studies and the results were considered inconclusive. The study would also look at all the health issues being examined in the estrogen-plus-progestin study; other types of cancer, hip fractures, stroke, blood clots, and the overall risk of death.

The estrogen-alone study included over 10,000 women who were 50 to 79 years of age and had had a hysterectomy. The women were randomly assigned to take either 0.625 milligrams per day of Premarin or a placebo. They all received the same close follow-up as the women in the estrogen-plus-progestin study.

In February of 2004, after almost seven years, the NIH decided to stop the study. Results up to that point indicated that ET had no affect on the risk of heart disease and actually increased the risk of stroke. The risk of stroke increased by 39 percent in women taking estrogen compared with women taking a placebo. The women taking estrogen also had a 33 percent increased risk of venous thrombosis, including a potentially fatal condition known as pulmonary embolism where a clot lodges in a vein in the lungs. Despite these increased risks, there was no difference in the overall risk of death in women taking estrogen.

What Nurses Know . . .

Statistical Significance

When we talk about something being significant in general terms we mean that it has importance, that it is meaningful. In research, significance has a different meaning. Statistical significance refers to whether or not study results are likely or unlikely to have occurred by chance. If results have statistical significance *then we can feel pretty confident that they are due to the treatment or intervention being studied and would not have just happened anyway. We are not 100 percent confident, there is always a chance of error. Studies usually use five percent (0.05) as the cutoff for* statistical significance. *This means that there is only a five percent chance (or* probability *in study language) that the results occurred by chance and a 95 percent chance that they are related to the treatment or intervention.*

In research, just because something is statistically significant does not mean that it is important. Some "true" differences found in studies may be so small or matter so little in a real life setting that they are not meaningful.

ET did not appear to have any affect on colorectal cancer, but it did appear to lower the risk for breast cancer, though the difference was too small to have statistical significance. There was also an increase in the risk of mild dementia in women over 65 years of age, but there again, the difference was too small to have statistical significance either.

ET was very effective in preventing hip and other fractures and in relieving hot flashes and night sweats. Similar to women taking estrogen-plus-progestin, women taking estrogen alone reported slight improvements in sleep, physical functioning, and body pain.

FOLLOW-UP

Researchers continued to monitor the women after the study ended. Three years after women in the study stopped taking hormones the increased risk of heart attacks, stroke, and blood clots all went away. So did the benefit of fewer fractures and less colorectal cancer. There continued to be an overall increased cancer risk in the women who took the hormones compared with women who took the placebo. There was also a higher rate of death from any cause in women who took the hormones compared with women who took the placebo.

Putting It All In Perspective

Women reacted with fear and dismay when the WHI findings came out. Millions abruptly stopped taking their hormones. Many women got their information only from news reports, which often led to a misunderstanding of the meaning of the results.

It is important to note that these results apply to a group, not to individuals. The risk to each individual woman for any of the outcomes, whether a heart attack or stroke or breast cancer, is very small. Hearing that your risk of having a serious health problem is 25 or 30 percent greater sounds scary. But most of these are rare problems in women to begin with. So even when the risk increases, it's still a very small risk.

It helps to understand what the increased risk means in real numbers. For instance, let's take a look at the actual number of women that would be affected by the increased risk of heart disease in the estrogen-plus-progestin study. The study found a 29 percent increased risk of heart attacks in women taking estrogen-plus-progestin. This works out to seven more heart attacks in 10,000 women taking estrogen-plus-progestin for a year. The numbers for the other events are about the same; eight more women out of 10,000 would have invasive breast cancer, eight more would have a stroke, and eight more would have a pulmonary embolism.

When the WHI researchers looked at the risks by age of the woman and timing of HT, they found that women who started HT early in menopause and before the age of 60 actually had no increased risk for heart disease. In fact, there appeared to be a protective effect when HT was started before the age of 60 and within 10 years of reaching menopause. When started during this time period in a woman's life, it appears to slow the buildup of plaque in the arteries of the heart.

Results of the WHI study do not necessarily apply to women who have premature menopause. The average age of the women in the WHI study was 63 to 64 years. This age group has a very different risk versus benefit profile from women 40 and younger. Women younger than 40 will experience many more years without the protective aspects of estrogen, while at the same time have not yet developed the cardiovascular and cancer risk factors that increase with age. Therefore, the potential for benefit is greater and the potential for risk is less. More research is needed on HT in this group of women. In the meantime, the potential risk versus benefit needs to be determined for each individual woman.

Recent research is building on and defining the knowledge gained from the WHI studies. We know more about how specific factors affect the risks. We have information that better allows each individual woman to make a decision based on her unique situation. It is becoming clearer that when treatment is individualized, short-term HT early in menopause is a safe beneficial option for many women.

The Bottom Line: Current Recommendations

The current expert consensus is that the benefits of HT outweigh the risks when it is started in selected younger women soon after they reach menopause. As women who have never used estrogen get older, and time passes since menopause, the risks begin to outweigh the benefits and worsen over time.

Currently, HT is FDA-approved for short-term use to relieve moderate to severe vasomotor symptoms (hot flashes and night sweats) and vaginal atrophy, and FDA-approved for long-term use for the prevention of osteoporosis.

Decisions about HT use must be made on an individual basis after a thorough review of the personal risk versus benefit profile for each woman.

You must think about what level of risk you are willing to accept and the potential benefits you can expect from HT. Then talk to your health care provider about your personal level of risk. You need to consider your current age, your age at menopause, how long ago you reached menopause, cause of menopause (natural or induced), previous use of hormones, current or past diseases, and presence of risk factors for cardiovascular diseases or cancer.

If you are over the age of 60 or 10 years postmenopausal and have not used HT since reaching menopause, you need to think extra carefully about starting hormone treatment for any reason. You will be at greater risk for heart attacks, stroke, blood clots, and breast cancer.

If you are younger than 40 it is usually considered safe and appropriate to use HT until the age of natural menopause (about 50). You may also need to use higher doses than women who are older than 50.

How long a woman stays on HT varies. The general rule is that you want to take the smallest effective dose for the shortest period of time. However, there are certain situations where a longer period

What Nurses Know...

To determine your benefit versus risk profile, review the following with your health care provider:

1. Age

2. Time since menopause

3. Previous use of hormones

4. Cause of menopause

5. Severity of hot flashes

6. Use of nonestrogen treatment for hot flashes

7. Personal and family history of heart disease

8. Presence of other heart disease risk factors such as high blood pressure, high cholesterol, or a sedentary lifestyle

9. History of a stroke

10. History of a blood clot

11. Breast cancer history in self or first-degree relative

12. Presence of blood clotting disorder

13. Mother, grandmother, or sisters with osteoporosis or fractures

14. Results of bone density testing

15. Use of nonestrogen treatment for osteoporosis

16. Smoking history or currently a smoker

of therapy is beneficial or needed. The North American Menopause Society (NAMS) recommends three actions when HT is used long term: (1) you must clearly understand the potential risks and benefits, (2) you should be on the lowest effective dose, and (3) there must be close follow-up by your health care provider.

There are certain situations where HT is *contraindicated* or should only be *used with caution.* If you have a history of breast cancer or currently have breast cancer; if you have blood clots or history of a blood clot (deep vein thrombosis or pulmonary embolism); or if you have had a stroke or heart attack within the past year, you definitely should NOT be on HT.

If you have any of the following you should not take estrogen products:

- Abnormal vaginal bleeding
- Untreated endometrial hyperplasia (thickened uterine lining)
- Any estrogen-dependent tumor
- Liver disease
- Any chance you could be pregnant

In addition, estrogen-plus-progestogen products should not be used if you have the following:

- Problem with kidney function (renal insufficiency)
- Adrenal insufficiency

What Nurses Know . . .

Contraindications Versus Use With Caution

There are certain situations when certain drugs or treatments should not be used. They may interact with other *medication you are taking or potentially worsen another medical condition you have. The two terms you will most often see used in this situation are "contraindicated" or "use with caution."*

Contraindicated *is the stronger term and means that you should not use that drug or treatment. That doesn't mean that a "contraindicated" drug or treatment is never used, but there better be a really good reason to do so. Remember, whenever medical treatment is done, the benefits have to outweigh the risks. If the risks are greater, as they would be if something is contraindicated, then the benefits have to be really significant to overcome that. There are some situations where a drug or treatment has an "absolute contraindication," meaning it should absolutely not be used because doing so puts the user at risk for serious injury or death.*

There are very few things that would justify your health care provider prescribing something for you that is contraindicated. If he or she does ask why and have a thorough talk about the risks.

Use with caution *means your health care provider needs to think twice about prescribing a drug or treatment and then follow up with you very carefully while it's being used. If you are on a medication that should be used with caution, then your health care provider needs to closely monitor the effects and possible side effects. This may mean additional tests, periodic blood work, and more frequent follow-up office visits.*

If you are taking any drugs or treatments that are contraindicated or should be used with caution, then make sure you know what kinds of symptoms you need to watch for and what kind of problems you need to follow up on.

Following is a summary of the current recommendations from NAMS and the American Association of Clinical Endocrinologists regarding HT. There are a few important rules that must be applied to every one of the recommendations:

- Each individual woman must undergo a thorough assessment to determine her personal risk versus benefit profile before using HT.
- Women and their health care providers should constantly reassess their risk versus benefit profile while on HT.
- HT should only be tried after other available options have been tried and failed or if other available options are inappropriate.
- HT should be used at the lowest effective dose for the shortest period of time necessary.

RECOMMENDATIONS

Hot Flashes and Night Sweats   HT is appropriate in selected woman during perimenopause and early menopause for relief of moderate to severe hot flashes. Use of transdermal forms should be considered, as there might be less risk of blood clots then with oral forms.

Vaginal Atrophy   HT is appropriate in selected woman during perimenopause and early menopause for relief of vaginal atrophy symptoms. Vaginal forms should be used when treatment is only for vaginal symptoms, as they have lower risks. (For further discussion of vaginal atrophy, see Chapter 5.)

Sexual Function   Use of local HT is appropriate in selected women for relief of painful intercourse caused by vaginal atrophy. It is not appropriate as the sole treatment of problems with sexual desire or response. (For further discussion of sexual function, see Chapter 5.)

Osteoporosis   Long-term hormone treatment is appropriate for prevention of osteoporosis in selected women with decreased bone mass when other therapies are not an option. It should be used soon after menopause. Women and their health care providers should periodically reevaluate the risk versus benefit of continued use over time. Ongoing use should be evaluated with the awareness that once treatment is stopped, the benefit disappears. (For further discussion of osteoporosis, see Chapter 6.)

Cardiovascular Disease   HT should not be used for the prevention of heart disease in women of any age. However, if a woman starts HT for symptom relief early in menopause, there does not appear to be an increased risk of cardiovascular disease. There is beginning to be evidence that starting estrogen-alone therapy early in menopause may decrease risk, but more studies are needed.

Breast Cancer   HT is contraindicated in women with known or suspected breast cancer or with a history of breast cancer. Women without a history of breast cancer need to discuss their personal risk versus benefit profile with their health care providers. Using HT for five years or more increases risk of breast cancer and is not recommended for most women.

Dementia   HT is not recommended for the prevention of dementia, including Alzheimer's disease, in women of any age. Findings of a few very small studies indicate that HT started immediately after a younger woman has her ovaries removed may improve memory. However, these studies do not provide enough strong evidence to recommend using HT for dementia prevention.

Depression   HT should not be used to treat depression in women of any age. Currently, there is mixed evidence regarding menopause and depression. Some evidence indicates that HT may have a positive effect on mood and behavior in menopausal women. However, it is not strong enough to support using HT to treat depression.

What Nurses Know...

Making a decision about HT is probably among the most important health care decisions you will make during your life. So take your time and prepare yourself. Think about what is important to you, your lifestyle, and your relationships. Think about how you view getting older. Talk to your friends. Read over this chapter carefully a few times. Take a look at the resources that follow.

You WILL make the right decision. Right for you; not for your sister or your best friend or your mother. And then you will go on to have the best possible next phase of your life.

Resources

Women's Health Initiative (WHI)
This NIH Web site has information on the WHI, a major 15-year research program looking at postmenopausal women. Click on the link on the right, NHLBI Postmenopausal Hormone Therapy, for comprehensive information on HT.
www.nhlbi.nih.gov/whi/

North American Menopause Society (NAMS)
NAMS is a nonprofit professional organization dedicated to promoting menopause-related health and quality of life. It does this through research, education, and resources for women and health care providers. The Web site has comprehensive information on menopause for women, as well as updated treatment guidelines and recommendations. Information is available in English, Spanish, and French.
www.menopause.org/

Facts About Menopausal Hormone Therapy
This fact sheet reviews the findings of the WHI study and provides easy-to-understand information about menopause, HT, and other ways to treat symptoms. It is published by the NIH and the National Heart, Lung, and Blood Institute.
www.nhlbi.nih.gov/health/women/pht_facts.pdf

National Cancer Institute (NCI)
The NCI Web site has a section on menopausal HT, with links to information on HT as it relates to cancer. There are three pages of information; click Next Section at the bottom of the page to move to pages 2 and 3.
www.cancer.gov/clinicaltrials/digest-postmenopausal-hormone-use

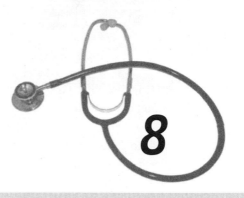

8

Using Hormone Therapy: The Practicalities

Hormone therapy (HT) is recommended when a clear need has been established. Treatment decisions will be based on what that need is, along with your personal health history and current health status, costs of various products, and personal choice. By now you should have had a thorough discussion of risks and benefits with your provider. Repeat that discussion periodically. Your risk versus benefit profile will change as time goes by. And so will what we know. We are constantly gaining new information about HT and you want to make sure your treatment continues to be based on the best and most up-to-date information.

Health Evaluation

Before you start HT you must have a complete health evaluation. You may already have done some of what this includes as part of your decision-making process. You will need to review your health history with your health care provider. It is very important to find out what risk factors you have for cardiovascular disease, blood clots, stroke, breast cancer, and osteoporosis.

Your health history includes your family medical history. If you don't know about your family history, this is the time to ask. Don't assume that because something has never been mentioned that it never happened.

Make sure you let your health care provider know about any alternative therapies you are on or have tried. This includes herbal products and dietary supplements. Some of these have active ingredients that may affect how you feel, interact with conventional hormone products, or impact your response to treatment.

Your health care provider may order a number of different tests, depending on your potential risk profile. For instance, if you have a family history of heart disease you may need a complete cardiac evaluation before starting HT. All women should have a mammogram if they have not had one within 12 months. Other tests that may be done include:

- Pap smear
- Blood tests to check lipid levels
- Pelvic ultrasound
- Breast ultrasound
- Bone density tests
- Electrocardiogram
- Treadmill cardiac stress test

BLOOD AND SALIVARY HORMONE LEVELS

Doing saliva or blood tests to find your hormone levels before starting treatment or to adjust your hormone treatment is not necessary or recommended. Many factors affect the hormone levels in your blood and your levels will differ from one day to another, and even within the same day. There is no evidence of any connection between hormone levels in your blood and menopausal symptoms or your response to treatment. Current best practice guidelines call for treatment to be based on symptom relief. You start on the lowest possible dose and it is adjusted upward until symptoms improve.

What Nurses Know...

In these days of 15-minute office visits, it's important to arrive for your evaluation prepared. Information you should gather about your health history includes:

- *History of breast cancer*

- *History of breast disease such as fibrocystic breast disease*

- *History of heart disease*

- *Age at first period and age at last period*

- *Any abnormal Pap smears or breast examinations*

- *Number of pregnancies and outcomes*

- *History of vascular disease such as deep vein thrombosis, a blood clot usually in the legs*

- *Use of oral contraceptive pills and any problems you had with them*

- *History of migraine headaches, especially those with aura*

- *Family history of breast cancer*

- *Family history of heart disease*

- *Family history of dementia*

- *Family history of osteoporosis*

If you have had any diagnostic testing done in the last 12 months bring a copy of the results with you

There is no scientific evidence to support the use of salivary testing. Current testing methods have not been found to be consistently accurate. Even if testing were accurate, we don't know what the optimum hormone levels are in postmenopausal women.

What Nurses Know...

Money Matters

Salivary testing is expensive. It can cost hundreds of dollars to have initial and follow-up tests done. Most insurance companies do not cover the cost of tests.

There is no one "normal" level that all women should aim for. Most medical experts strongly advise against salivary testing.

Using Hormone Therapy

Hormone therapy is available in systemic and local formulations. Systemic forms include oral (swallowed) and transdermal forms (skin patches, creams, and gels). Vaginal estrogen products are topical agents that work locally rather than systemically.

Topical vaginal estrogen is the best option if you just need relief of vaginal symptoms. Medications that are systemic are metabolized throughout the body and so have effects, sometimes unwanted, on areas unrelated to the problem for which you are taking the medication. When topical agents are used many side effects are avoided or minimized, or larger doses of the medication can be used more safely.

Transdermal products are not a local treatment even though they are applied topically. They are absorbed slowly through the skin into the systemic circulation. Because they are a systemic agent they have the same potential for side effects and risk factors as HT taken orally (except for Menostar, a very-low-dose skin patch). However, there is some evidence that using transdermal products carries less risk of blood clots and strokes than oral medications. This is probably related to its not being

What Nurses Know...

Systemic products come in different modes of delivery, so don't be misled into thinking that just because something is not in pill form or taken orally that it is not a systemic acting agent. For instance, skin patches are designed to deliver a high enough dose to act systemically.

metabolized through the liver before reaching the blood stream, like oral medications are.

Finding the HT regimen that is best for you may be a process of trial and error. There are many different hormone products available and each individual woman may react differently to them. Let your health care provider know if you are having unpleasant side effects or the therapy isn't giving you the relief you need.

Be patient and persistent about finding the right drug and dose for you. There are a number of options available. You can adjust the dose, try a different type of estrogen or progestogen, change the scheduling of an estrogen-plus-progestogen regimen (i.e., from continuous to intermittent or vice versa), or switch to a skin patch. All changes should be done with the guidance of your health care provider.

If you still have your uterus, you will be put on an estrogen-plus-progestogen regimen to prevent the buildup of the endometrium (uterine lining) that can lead to endometrial cancer. Unless you are only using vaginal estrogen, very little estrogen gets into the circulation with most vaginal estrogen products. If you are using one of the stronger vaginal preparations, your health care provider may decide to add a progestogen product to protect the uterus.

What Nurses Know...

Tips for Taking Medication

• Take medications at the same time every day. Set an alarm on your watch or cell phone, or link it to an activity such as brushing your teeth or having your morning coffee.

• Refill prescriptions before you run out. Put a reminder on your calendar or program it into your phone.

• Keep an updated list of your medications. Bring the list, or even better, the actual medications, to every visit you have with a health care provider. Include all over-the-counter medicine, supplements, vitamins, herbal preparations, and topical products.

• Do not adjust your medications without talking to your health care provider.

• Do not stop a medication without talking to your health care provider. Some medications need to be tapered down when you stop using them.

• Tell your health care provider if you drink grapefruit juice. Grapefruit juice affects the metabolism of many drugs.

If you have had a hysterectomy, then you will be put on estrogen alone. The only reason to take a progestogen is to prevent endometrial cancer. If you don't have a uterus then you don't need to worry about endometrial cancer, so you can avoid the risks and side effects related to progestogen use.

What Nurses Know...

If you are on thyroid medication for hypothyroid (low thyroid) you should have your thyroid level checked after you start taking any product containing estrogen. You may have to increase your dose when you're on estrogen therapy (ET).

TAKING ESTROGEN-PLUS-PROGESTOGEN

Progesterone levels control the shedding of the endometrium during the menstrual cycle. The addition of a progestogen to ET keeps the lining of the endometrium from thickening too much (endometrial hyperplasia), which can lead to endometrial cancer. Most women will experience some withdrawal bleeding when using an estrogen-plus-progestogen product, at least early on in the therapy. Usually bleeding decreases or even stops altogether after a year or so.

There are a number of different options for taking estrogen-plus-progestogen: continuous-combined, continuous-cycle, cyclic,

What Nurses Know...

When you start using a progestogen you will have withdrawal bleeding similar to having a period. Bleeding should not be heavy or prolonged. Report any unusual bleeding to your health care provider right away. Also let them know if there is an increase in amount, frequency, or duration of bleeding after you have been on the product for a period of time.

intermittent-combined, and long-cycle therapy are the most common methods. Deciding which to use is mostly a matter of personal choice based on convenience. The most important consideration for most women is the extent of withdrawal bleeding associated with each method.

In *continuous-combined* therapy you take a combination of estrogen-plus-progestogen everyday. This can be done in the form of a combination pill or a skin patch (transdermal). There is less bleeding with this option; 60 percent of women who use it will not have any bleeding. After a year, most women (90%) will not have any bleeding at all.

In *continuous-cycle* therapy you take estrogen everyday and add a progestogen for 10 to 14 days every month. With this method, 80 percent of women bleed when the progestogen is stopped but over time the bleeding lessens, and after about a year it usually stops completely.

If you choose *cyclic therapy* you will take estrogen for 25 days each month and add a progestogen for the last 10 to 14 days. Then you go for three days without taking either estrogen or a progestogen. You will bleed when you stop the progestogen. Many women complain of hot flashes during the days they are off estrogen. This is the least popular option and is used infrequently.

● ●

Progestogen Products

Following are progestogen-alone products available in the United States:

Oral Progestin Tablets:
Provera—medroprogesterone acetate
Micronor, Nor-QD, generics—norethindrone
Ovrette—norgestrel

Oral Progesterone Capsules:
Prometrium—progesterone

Vaginal Progesterone Gel:
Prochieve—progesterone

If you choose *intermittent-combined* therapy, you will take estrogen every day of the month and take a progestogen in cycles of three days on and three days off throughout the month. Women using this option usually have a bleeding pattern similar to that of women using continuous-combined therapy.

Long-cycle therapy is a newer combined therapy option. You take estrogen every day, but can go three to six months in between progestogen doses. More research is needed about the effects of long-term therapy on the endometrium and other risks related to HT.

Drospirenone differs from other progestogen products in that it is a synthetic progesterone combined with spironolactone, a diuretic. Spironolactone is a potassium-sparing diuretic. That

* *

Estrogen-Plus-Progestogen Products

Following are estrogen-plus-progestogen products available in the United States:

Continuous-Combined Products
Tablets:
Prempro—conjugated estrogens and medroxyprogesterone acetate
Premplus—conjugated estrogens and medroxyprogesterone acetate
Femhrt—ethinyl estradiol
Activella—17beta-estradiol and norethindrone acetate
Angeliq—17beta-estradiol and drospirenone
Skin Patch:
CombiPatch—17beta-estradiol and norethindrone acetate
Climara Pro—17beta-estradiol and levonorgestrel

Continuous-Cycle Products
Tablets:
Premphase—conjugated estrogens and medroxyprogesterone acetate
Skin Patch:
Estracomb—17beta-estradiol and norethindrone acetate

Intermittent-Combined Products
Tablets:
Prefest—17beta-estradiol and norgestimate
Skin Patch:
Not available

means it gets rid of water but not potassium, so when taking it you must avoid eating large quantities of foods that are high in potassium. Elevated potassium levels can be harmful. Foods high in potassium include potatoes, citrus fruits, bananas, and tomatoes. You don't have to avoid them completely; you just don't want to overdo it. Check the ingredients of vitamin-enriched drinks and vitamin tablets for potassium, as well.

Products containing drospirenone should not be used if you have kidney problems, especially if you're also taking certain medications, including nonsteroidal anti-inflammatory drugs (NSAIDs) like ibuprofen (Advil, Motrin) or the blood pressure medicines angiotensin-converting enzyme (ACE) inhibitors (Lotension, Captopril, Vasotec, Altace), and angiotension II receptor blockers (Avapro, Cozaar, Diovan).

TAKING ESTROGEN ALONE

Estrogen products come in a number of different forms. The most popular are oral tablets, followed by transdermal patches. There are also transdermal gels and creams that are applied directly on the skin.

Transdermal patches store a supply of estrogen in the adhesive layer of the patch. The estrogen is released continuously and slowly into your circulation. Most are changed once or twice a

What Nurses Know...

Most salt substitutes contain potassium. Do not use them if you are taking drospirenone.

If you are restricting salt (sodium) in your diet try using other spices to season your food. Garlic, ground pepper, tarragon, oregano, nutmeg, and cinnamon are some excellent choices to add flavor and zing to dishes.

What Nurses Know . . .

Tips for using skin patches

- *Remove the old patch before applying the new one. Do this every time so you develop a routine and are less likely to forget to remove the old patch*

- *Change the site every time you change the patch*

- *Do not apply to irritated skin*

- *Never cut the patch with scissors*

- *Do not apply extra patches to try and catch up on missed doses*

- *Fold the used patch with sticky sides together and **throw it away where children and pets can't get it***

week. You can bathe and swim with the patch on, though it is a good idea to always check that it is still in place afterward.

Creams and gels are applied once a day to an arm or leg, or both arms or legs. They dry quickly and are invisible and odorless once dry. The cream or gel is absorbed into the outer layer of skin from where it is absorbed slowly into your system over the next 24 hours. There is also a topical spray that works the same way as creams and gels.

If you are using HT only for relief of symptoms related to vaginal atrophy, such as dryness and painful sexual intercourse, then you should be using a local vaginal preparation, not a systemic product. Combination therapy with a progestogen is not needed when these products are used. They are also safe for long-term use, and in women over 60 years of age or far out from menopause.

What Nurses Know...

If using creams or gel products, make sure you wash your hands well with soap and water after applying the product. Medication left on your hands can get passed on to others that you come into contact with.

There is one vaginal product (Femring) that is strong enough to have a systemic effect. Unlike other vaginal products, it is approved for treatment of hot flashes as well as vaginal atrophy. If you have an intact uterus and are using this product, you need to be taking a progestogen as well.

Side Effects of Estrogen and Estrogen-Progestogen Therapy

Fluid retention and bloating, breast tenderness, headaches, mood swings...sound familiar? If you took "the pill" or had pre-menstrual syndrome (PMS), you will recognize many of the side effects caused by HT. They are very similar. This time, though, you do not need to suffer through them.

Most side effects can be relieved with changes to your hormone regimen. If you have side effects, talk to your health care provider about adjusting your dose, or changing the hormone product or scheduling method you are using. Usually one or a combination of these strategies will take care of any side effects.

If you continue to have side effects, there are four lifestyle changes that can help with all of the side effects listed above. All of these changes are beneficial for your general health, as well.

1. Restrict salt intake
2. Drink plenty of water

3. Reduce caffeine
4. Exercise regularly

Some women on oral estrogen have problems with nausea. If this happens to you, try taking the tablets with food. If you take it with food just before bedtime you may sleep right through the nausea (this probably is not the best plan if you have insomnia).

● ●

Estrogen Products

Following are estrogen-alone products available in the United States:

Oral Products
Premarin—conjugated estrogens
Cenestin, Enjuvia—synthetic-conjugated estrogens
Menest—esterified estrogens
Estrace—17beta-estradiol
Femtrace—estradiol acetate
Ortho-Est—estropipate

Transdermal Products
Alora, Climara, Esclim, Menostar, Vivelle, Vivelle-Dot—17beta-estradiol matrix patch
Estraderm—17beta-estradiol reservoir patch

Topical Products
EstroGel 0.06 percent, Elestrin 0.06 percent, Divigel 0.1 percent—17beta-estradiol transdermal gel
Estrasorb—17beta-estradiol topical emulsion
Evamist—17beta-estradiol transdermal spray

Vaginal Products
Creams:
Estrace Vaginal Cream—17beta-estradiol
Premarin Vaginal Cream—conjugated estrogens
Rings:
Estring—17beta-estradiol
Femring—estradiol acetate
Tablets:
Vagifem—estradiol hemihydrate

What Nurses Know...

Some foods have a natural diuretic effect and can help relieve water retention and bloating. They include:

Celery

Onion

Eggplant

Asparagus

Watermelon

Apple cider vinegar

Cranberry

Natural herbal diuretics can be helpful as well. They include:

Chicory

Dandelion

Parsley

Ginger

Juniper

Some women who use the skin patches have a problem with skin irritation from the adhesive on the patch. You can try moving the patch to a different area or switching to a patch with a different adhesive. Make sure the skin is clean and dry before applying the patch and change the site every time you change the patch. If the problem continues you may have to switch to a cream or gel.

Bioidentical and Custom-Compounded Hormones: What Are They Really?

More and more women are turning to bioidentical and custom-compounded hormone products. When the Women's Health Initiative study results came out (see Chapter 7), many women reacted with fear and distrust of established HT. Recent endorsement by celebrities has brought even more attention to these products. The belief that personalized "natural" products are different from conventional products and hence better for you has become commonplace.

It is difficult to separate the hype from the facts. The medical community has spoken out on the issue but women have lost trust in the medical community and few listen. Adding to the confusion is the frequent use of the terms *bioidentical*, *custom-compounded*, and *natural* as if they all mean the same thing.

Bioidentical means that a hormone is the same or very similar to hormones made by your body. Bioidentical and natural are not the same, though the terms are often used as if they are. *Natural* means something that comes from nature, whether it is from a plant, animal, or mineral. The plants most commonly used in bioidentical hormone products are Mexican yams and soy. Some hormone products are made from natural substances but are not bioidentical. Cenestin, for example, is made from plants but it is not structurally the same as endogenous estrogen.

What Nurses Know...

Money Matters

Custom-compounded products can be expensive and many insurance companies do not cover them.

Custom-compounded bioidentical products are individualized hormone products made to order. They contain a combination of hormones derived from plant sources that most commonly include estrogen, progesterone, testosterone, or dehydroepiandrosterone (DHEA). Health care providers write a prescription for a certain combination and dosage of hormones and a compounding pharmacy makes the product.

There are no good studies that have examined the safety or effectiveness of custom-compounded bioidentical products. The few studies that have been conducted have major flaws and the results are not reliable. There is certainly no evidence to support claims that these products are safer or more effective than conventional hormones.

The promotion of "natural" custom-compounded bioidentical hormones as superior to conventional hormones is usually based on two primary claims. First, "natural" custom-compounded bioidentical hormones are identical copies of the hormones your body makes, so they are safer than conventional hormones. Second, they are a "natural" product versus a "synthetic" product created by a drug company. These claims are misleading and there is no evidence to support them. Let's take a look at each of them.

Bioidentical hormones are identical copies of the hormones your body makes, so they are safer.

Custom-compounded and "natural" hormones are not unique because they are bioidentical. There are many prescription hormones that are bioidentical as well. If an estrogen product is made of 17beta-estradiol it is bioidentical. If a progestogen is made of micronized progesterone it is bioidentical. Nor are custom-compounded and "natural" bioidentical hormones more natural than conventional hormones. Many conventional hormones are made from the same plants as "natural" bioidentical products.

They are a "natural" product versus a "synthetic" product created by a drug company. All hormone products are synthetic in the truest sense of the word. Yam and soy plants do not contain estrogen. It is *synthesized* from a substance in the plants called diosgensin. Once a compound becomes estrogen, your body uses it the same way regardless of how it started out. There may be differences based on the type of estrogen—estradiol or estrone, for instance. There may also be differences in the absorption based on the substance the estrogen is held in or the route used to get it into circulation. In fact, one of the problems with custom-compounded supplements is the lack of consistency in their delivery and absorption.

If conventional hormones are contraindicated, then you should not be using any hormone product. The risks of exposure to hormones are the same whether they are bioidentical or not. In fact, "natural" bioidentical hormones can be more risky than prescription hormones because they are not regulated by the Food and Drug Administration (FDA). This means that ingredients and doses are not monitored for consistency and purity.

We need good research on custom-compounded and other "natural" bioidentical hormone products. Currently we don't know their true safety or effectiveness or how they compare with

What Nurses Know ...

Beware of articles and Internet sites that promote hormone products. HT is a multibillion dollar business. This includes prescription drugs and so-called "natural products," as well. Many so-called health articles are actually advertisements in disguise.

If you get to the end of an article or Web page and the writer encourages you to buy a product, it is likely the article was written specifically to market the product and is biased. Get your information from Web sites and articles written solely to provide information. There are Resources included at the end of this chapter for reputable sources.

conventional hormone products. Future studies may find there are some advantages to using them over conventional hormones. We also need to establish mechanisms for close monitoring of dose consistency. This does not mean that every custom-compounded or other "natural" bioidentical product will be the same dosage. It means that a particular stated dose is the same in every product, every time. So if you are supposed to get five milligrams, you always get five milligrams. Studies show that this is often not the case.

There are isolated cases where women who do not do well on conventional hormone products may benefit from custom-compounded hormones. This is something that needs to be discussed in-depth with your health care provider. However, for now most women are better off using conventional hormones; they have been extensively studied and are monitored by the FDA for product safety, dose, and purity.

Stopping Hormone Therapy

My gyn put me on estrogen after I had a total hysterectomy but I took myself off. I tapered off and for the first year after that I was fine. But the next year the hot flashes were horrendous!   SUE

When you stop HT the benefits stop along with it. If you are taking it for the relief of hot flashes and night sweats you are likely to start having them again. If you are taking it for prevention of osteoporosis, within five years of stopping therapy your risk of fracture will reach the same level as women who did not use HT.

Some women have found that tapering off of HT slowly helps. However, studies don't show any difference in symptoms between women who taper off and women who stop abruptly. Many women find the returning symptoms intolerable and end up restarting HT. Make sure you talk to your health care provider if you decide to restart therapy so appropriate follow-up is in place.

When you are ready to stop HT discuss it with your health care provider. It may be helpful to start a program of alternative strategies to relieve hot flashes (for more on these see Chapter 3)

while you taper off. Do not take estrogen-like products while you are tapering off of HT. Supplements and other "natural" products are not regulated and the strength can be inconsistent. You could be wreaking havoc on your hormonal balance, the last thing you need as your body is adjusting to the withdrawal of exogenous hormones.

Resources

MayoClinic.com
The Mayo Clinic menopause section includes information on HT. Click on the *In-Depth* tab and go to Treatments and drugs. www.mayoclinic.com/health/menopause/DS00119

MedlinePlus
This government Web site is a service of the National Institutes of Health. Scroll down to the section on Treatment to find links to information on HT. Information is available in 12 languages. www.nlm.nih.gov/medlineplus/menopause.html

North American Menopause Society (NAMS)
NAMS is a nonprofit professional organization dedicated to promoting the menopause-related health and quality of life. There is a chapter on HT in the Menopause Guidebook. Go to *For Consumers* and click on Menopause Guidebook on the right. You can download individual chapters. www.menopause.org/

International Academy of Compounding Pharmacists
The Web site for this nonprofit organization offers a compounding pharmacist locator. www.iacprx.org

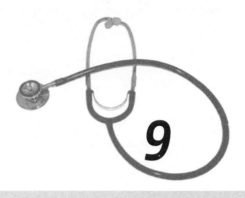

9

Health and Harmony

As we get older our risk for certain health conditions increases. Your cholesterol and blood pressure creep up, increasing your risk of heart disease. The rate of breast cancer and colon cancer increases. The loss of estrogen at menopause adds to these risks.

You are not at the mercy of age and hormones. There are things you can do to optimize your health after menopause. Eating a low-fat diet, maintaining your ideal body weight (IBW), and exercising regularly are one set of actions essential to good health. The other is health screening. Following is a review of current recommendations for preventive health screening in women in the menopausal years.

Health Screening

BREAST CANCER

There is probably no other diagnosis that strikes fear in the minds of women in the United States like that of breast cancer.

For good reason—breast cancer is the most common cancer and the second leading cause of cancer-related deaths in women. And for most women, breasts are not merely another part of the body; they embody sexuality, femininity, motherhood, and nurturance.

What Nurses Know...

There was a lot of backlash when new U.S. Preventive Services Task Force breast screening recommendations came out in 2009. It may be helpful to understand how health screening recommendations are decided on.

Health screening recommendations are based on 10 criteria known as the Wilson-Jungner criteria.

1. *Condition is an important health problem*

2. *Early treatment is available*

3. *Diagnostic and treatment facilities are available*

4. *Condition is detectable at an early stage*

5. *Suitable test is available*

6. *Test is acceptable to the public*

7. *Natural course of condition is well understood*

8. *There is an agreed-upon policy on whom to treat*

9. *Costs of screening and treatment are economically balanced in relation to cost of medical care overall*

10. *Detecting the condition should be a continual process, not a one-time project*

In 2009 the United States Preventive Services Task Force (USPSTF) changed the breast screening recommendations, causing an uproar in the process. The biggest changes, and the ones that caused the controversy, recommended that women with average risk undergo annual routine mammography starting at the age of 50 instead of 40 and that from age 50 to 75 they should have routine screening every two years instead of every one to two years. The decision was likely based on the fact that the benefit of screening was small in women younger than 50. You only need to screen 1,339 women between 50 and 74 years of age to save one life, but 1,904 women would need to be screened in the 40- to 49-year age group.

Of course, if that one woman is you or someone you love, you probably think it is worth it. Unfortunately, it is not that simple. Decisions about screening recommendations are based on population health, not individuals. Health care resources are limited and need to be used where they will provide the most benefit. Also, the benefit of screening has to outweigh the risks, and there are risks to mammography screening. Mammography screening exposes all women to radiation, and most women experience pain during the procedure. There is a high number of false positive readings; it is estimated that half of all women who have at least 10 mammograms during their lives will have at least one false positive result. These women go through undue fear and anxiety, sometimes lasting long after they find out there is really nothing wrong. Others undergo unnecessary procedures, including surgery, due to erroneous results or the finding of an abnormality that never would have caused a problem in the long run.

Currently, the American Cancer Society still recommends annual routine mammography for women beginning at the age of 40. The USPSTF modified their recommendation to state that women in their 40s should make an individual decision about routine screening based on how they feel about the risks and benefits.

Keep in mind that both these recommendations are for women at *average* risk of breast cancer. Those with increased risk need to start screening earlier. If you have a first-degree relative (mother, daughter, or sister) with a history of breast cancer, or if you have had radiation treatment to the chest area you need to be extra vigilant about breast cancer screening. You should start annual screenings earlier and never miss your yearly mammogram.

Performing breast self-examination (BSE) is no longer recommended. If you do BSE, make sure you get instructions on the correct technique from your health care provider. BSE is not a substitute for mammogram or clinical breast examination. An annual clinical breast examination (performed by your health care provider) is still recommended.

PAP SMEARS

After you turn 30 you only need to have a Pap smear every three years if you have had three normal results in a row. After the age of 70 you do not need to have a Pap smear if you have had three normal results in a row and no abnormal results in the previous 10 years.

OVARIAN CANCER

Screening for ovarian cancer using ultrasound or checking the level of CA-125 in the blood is not currently recommended. CA-125 is a tumor marker, a substance found in higher levels in cancer cells than in other cells. Studies find that many unnecessary surgeries are performed when either method is used, and even when ovarian cancer was found as a result, it was already in a late stage.

COLORECTAL CANCER

Women who have average risk of colorectal cancer should begin screening at 50 years of age. There are a number of options recommended by the American Cancer Society. You must follow up with a colonoscopy if you have a positive result with any of the other options.

- *Colonoscopy* every 10 years. This test uses a lighted flexible tube to examine the entire colon (large intestine). You have to do a "bowel prep" beforehand to clean out the colon. Most people consider this the worst part of the procedure. You will be on a liquid diet for one or two days before the test and then take a strong laxative the night before. The laxative causes frequent, often forceful, diarrhea. You may also need to take enemas the morning of the test. The test is performed under "conscious sedation"; you are awake but drowsy. The medication used also causes amnesia, so even though you are awake you will have no memory of the procedure.

• *CT colonoscopy* every five years. This is also called a virtual colonoscopy. It uses computerized axial tomography (CAT) scanning to create images of the inside of the colon. The preparation for the test is the same as for a colonoscopy.

• *Flexible sigmoidoscopy* every five years. This test uses a lighted flexible tube to examine the lower third of the colon. It does not require anesthesia or sedatives, though some people prefer to take a mild sedative before the test. Usually one or two enemas the morning of the procedure are all that is needed to clean out the bowel to prepare for the test.

• *Double-contrast barium enema* every five years. In this test, contrast material (barium) is inserted into the colon through a tube placed in the anus. The barium is then removed so that only a thin layer remains. X-rays are then taken of the colon. This test also requires the same bowel preparation as a colonoscopy.

CHOLESTEROL

Cholesterol has a bad reputation but it actually has important functions in the body. It makes up the lining of all cell walls, is a building block for certain hormones, and protects peripheral nerves. The body, though, only needs a small amount of this waxy, fatty substance and the trouble arises when you have too much. When cholesterol levels get too high the excess sticks to the walls of your arteries, causing a plaque that narrows the vessel and blocks blood flow. Complete blockage of one of the arteries that supplies blood to the heart muscle will cause a heart attack. Sometimes you will have warnings that this is happening as the vessel narrows over time, but it also can happen suddenly if a blood clot gets stuck on plaque that has formed.

The liver makes about 75 percent of your body's cholesterol supply; the rest comes from the food you eat. Genetics is a factor in how much cholesterol your liver makes. You control how much you consume in food.

You should have your cholesterol levels checked every five years unless you have risk factors for heart disease. Risk factors are smoking, high blood pressure (hypertension), and a family history of early coronary heart disease (atherosclerosis or heart attack before age 55 in men, and 65 in women). If you have any of these risk factors, or previous cholesterol tests were abnormal or close to abnormal, than you will need to have your levels checked more often.

Cholesterol screening is done with a blood test called a lipoprotein panel. There are four types of cholesterol measured with a lipoprotein panel: total cholesterol, low-density lipoproteins (LDLs), high-density lipoproteins (HDLs), and triglycerides.

Total cholesterol is simply a measurement of the overall cholesterol in your blood. High total cholesterol levels can be an

What Nurses Know . . .

Being thin doesn't guarantee low cholesterol levels. People who are overweight do tend to have higher cholesterol levels, but thin people can have high levels as well. Even if you are at your IBW, genes and diet will have an effect on your cholesterol.

Cholesterol Levels

Total Cholesterol
<200 Desirable
200–239 Borderline high
≥240 High

LDL Cholesterol
<100 Optimal
100–129 Near optimal
130–159 Borderline high
160–189 High
≥190 Very high

HDL Cholesterol
<40 Low
≥60 High (desirable)

Triglycerides
<150 Normal
150–199 Borderline high
200–499 High
≥500 Very high

indication of cardiovascular risk. More important is how that level is divided between LDLs and HDLs.

LDL is the "bad cholesterol" that causes the buildup of plaque on blood vessel walls. The lower your LDL level, the lower your risk of cardiovascular disease, including heart attack and stroke.

HDL is the "good cholesterol" that helps sweep up excess cholesterol along blood vessel walls and carries it back to the liver where the digestive system takes over and gets rid of it. HDL also helps prevent blood vessel constriction and injury. The higher your HDL level, the lower your risk of cardiovascular disease.

Triglycerides function differently from LDL and HDL cholesterol. It is not used as a building block for cell walls and hormones. It is the fat your body uses for energy. Your body turns extra calories into triglycerides. When you consistently eat more than you need for energy, your triglyceride level will go up.

Staying Healthy

CARDIOVASCULAR HEALTH

Cardiovascular disease is the number one killer of women older than 55 years. Menopause causes changes that can increase your risk of cardiovascular disease. The shift in fat to the abdominal area and increased weight overall can lead to high blood pressure, abnormal cholesterol levels, and insulin resistance. Insulin resistance raises the level of insulin in the blood because cells aren't using it the way they ordinarily would. Higher blood insulin causes your body to retain sodium (salt) and fluid, raising blood pressure even more. There are also changes in the functioning of blood vessels themselves. They become less flexible and less responsive to increased demands. Increased inflammatory changes in the blood vessel lining amplify the danger of high cholesterol, increasing plaque buildup.

Controlling your blood pressure and cholesterol levels are essential for cardiovascular health after menopause. Lifestyle measures are the first, and often only, measures needed. Refer to the section on weight control in Chapter 10 for more information on diet and exercise, key components of cardiovascular health.

Blood Pressure   You should have your blood pressure checked annually, unless it is high or borderline high. Then you will need more frequent checks. The desired range for the top number, called the systolic pressure, is from 90 to 120; the bottom number, the diastolic, should be from 60 to 80. If either of those two numbers starts creeping above those values you need to take action. High blood pressure has actually been found to be more dangerous in women than in men, causing almost double the risk of cardiovascular disease than it does in men.

Weight loss, exercise, and diet changes often are all you need to keep your blood pressure where you want it. The first step is to lower your salt intake. A 2010 study in the *New England Journal of Medicine* found that decreasing salt intake by 1,200 milligrams a day would cut in half new cases of coronary

What Nurses Know...

A number of factors can raise your blood pressure temporarily. A stressful event, having just exercised, a sleepless night, or certain medications such as over-the-counter (OTC) cold medicines can result in a high reading. Some people have white-coat syndrome, a condition where just being in the provider's office raises their blood pressure. If your blood pressure is high it should be checked on two or three different occasions before you're diagnosed with hypertension.

heart disease and also almost halve the number of deaths from stroke and heart attacks each year. If you are overweight, start a healthy weight-loss diet; even losing just five pounds can make a difference.

You should also limit alcohol to one drink a day and avoid caffeine. Getting adequate sleep, seven to eight hours a night, and stress management will help control your blood pressure as well. Alternative therapies like yoga, meditation, deep breathing exercises, and biofeedback can make a difference.

If your blood pressure is consistently over 140/90 despite lifestyle changes, you will need to start medication. Sometimes a diuretic (water pill) is enough, other times you will need antihypertensive medications. You and your health care provider will decide what is best for you.

Cholesterol

After menopause my cholesterol went up sky high. It went from 180 to 280 in the first year. For 6 months I tried everything—stepped up exercise, ate really well. But finally I had to go on medication, just a low dose though. Now it's down to 160.   LIZ

Medications to Lower Cholesterol

There are a number of medications available to lower LDLs and triglycerides. Your provider will choose the best one for you based on your blood test results. Some medications are more effective at lowering LDLs, whereas others are better at lowering triglycerides. Women actually respond to lipid-lowering agents better than men.

Elevated cholesterol needs to be treated promptly and aggressively; even slightly abnormal levels increase a woman's risk for having a heart attack. Aggressive doesn't necessarily mean medication. Elevated LDLs and triglycerides can be treated first with dietary changes, lowering fat intake and increasing fiber intake, and increased physical activity. If that is not successful then cholesterol-lowering medication is needed.

Raising low HDL levels is more difficult than lowering LDL and triglyceride levels.

Exercise is the most effective way to elevate your HDL levels. Diet has only limited effect on HDL levels. Eating a low-fat diet that includes foods that contain omega-3 fatty acids, salmon is one of the best sources, is considered the most effective for raising HDL. Moderate alcohol consumption, one to two drinks a day, will also increase HDL levels. (It also lowers triglycerides and improves insulin sensitivity.) There are no medications that are specifically designed to increase HDL levels, but fibrate drugs have been found to have a positive effect. All of these measures will only have a modest effect at increasing HDL levels, but even a modest increase will help decrease cardiovascular risk, especially when combined with a lower LDL level.

Tobacco Use If you are a smoker, quit. Smoking triples your risk of dying of heart disease. Quitting won't be easy; tobacco is one of the most highly addictive drugs there is. If you are ready to quit and are having difficulty, talk to your provider about trying the medication bupropion, sold as Zyban or Wellbutrin. It is an antidepressant that for unknown reasons has been found to decrease the desire to smoke in people who want to quit. The use of nicotine patches is helpful in overcoming the physical dependence on nicotine. Nicotine patches can be used alone or in combination with bupropion.

ABNORMAL UTERINE BLEEDING

After menopause ANY vaginal bleeding is abnormal. It's that simple. If you have not had a period for more than 12 months and you have any vaginal bleeding, even spotting, even if it goes away, get to your gynecologist to get checked. At the very least you will need an ultrasound. Bleeding after menopause may be a sign of endometrial cancer.

It is not always cancer; in fact, only one out of 10 cases ends up to be cancer. Most of the time (about 7 out of 10) it is caused by endometrial atrophy (thinning of the endometrium). Other possible causes are polyps (noncancerous growths on the lining of the uterus), endometrial hyperplasia (thickening of the lining of the uterus), infection, and estrogen therapy. Whatever the cause, it is *always* something that needs to be addressed, not ignored.

URINARY HEALTH

> *I had stress incontinence after menopause. My bladder is extremely dropped. It was a big problem for awhile, but I stepped up the Kegel exercises big time and I really don't have a problem anymore, though I do have to empty my bladder frequently.* SUSAN

It is estimated that up to 60 percent of women will have mild incontinence as they get older, and about five percent will have severe problems. It is thought that decreasing estrogen levels during perimenopause is a factor in the development or worsening of incontinence, though some studies suggest that it is aging, not menopause, that is the prime culprit. Though poor urinary health doesn't pose the life-threatening risks that poor cardiovascular health does, it has a major impact on quality of life. The two most common types of urinary incontinence in women are stress incontinence and urge incontinence, also called overactive bladder. Some women will have a combination of both types.

Stress incontinence is the involuntary leakage of urine with actions that increase pressure on the bladder, like coughing, sneezing, heavy lifting, and laughing. It is caused by weakened bladder muscles. Women who have had multiple births are more prone to stress incontinence.

Urge incontinence happens when the urge to void comes on without warning. Suddenly you have to go, NOW! Urge incontinence can be caused by a urinary tract infection, medications that irritate the bladder, diseases of the nervous system, or neurological conditions like Parkinson's or Alzheimer's disease. Often there is no known cause.

The first thing you want to do is get checked for a urinary tract infection, especially if the urinary incontinence came on suddenly or worsened quickly. Treating the infection may be all you need to take care of the problem. If you are overweight, losing weight can lessen or even eliminate problems with incontinence. Other factors that will increase your risk of incontinence are anxiety and a diagnosis of diabetes.

What Nurses Know...

Drinking cranberry juice can help maintain urinary health. It acidifies the urine and prevents bacteria from sticking to the bladder walls.

If you are taking blood thinners (warfarin, Coumadin) talk to your health care provider first. Drinking large amounts of cranberry juice has been found to cause bleeding problems in people taking these medications.

Kegel exercises are very effective for strengthening the muscles of the pelvic floor and improving incontinence. They have the added benefit of increasing sexual pleasure for many women. However, they will only be effective if you do them correctly. You want to make sure that you are contracting the right muscles.

To learn which muscles to contract, you should practice stopping the flow of urine after you've started to void. Only do this to locate the muscles! If you perform Kegel exercises repeatedly when your bladder is full you can actually end up weakening your pelvic floor muscles. Another option to locate the right muscles is to insert a finger into your vagina and squeeze the muscles around it. If you are contracting the right muscles you will feel your vagina tighten around your finger and the floor of your pelvis lift.

Once you've got the technique you should contract the muscles, hold for four seconds, and relax for four seconds. Repeat this action 10 times in a row and do it at least three times a day. The great thing is that you can do them anywhere, anytime.

ORAL HEALTH

Good dental hygiene takes on even more importance as you get older. Our mouth tends to be drier, which increases your risk for caries (cavities) since saliva plays an important role in ongoing cleansing of your teeth. Menopause also increases your risk for tooth loss. This is probably related to osteoporosis in the jaw bones that support the teeth. As bones weaken, the teeth can become loose. It is also thought that lack of estrogen decreases the ability of gingival and periodontal tissue to respond to inflammation. If you aren't already, now is the time to get rigorous about brushing, flossing, and getting regular dental cleanings and checkups.

Burning Mouth Syndrome   If you feel like your mouth is on fire for no reason, you are not imaging things—you may be suffering from burning mouth syndrome. Burning mouth syndrome is just what it sounds like—a burning pain on the tongue and mouth, usually absent at night and worsening over the course of the day. It's usually accompanied by dryness and changes in taste. There is no apparent cause for the burning and we have yet to figure out what is happening to cause the sensation. Ninety percent of cases are in perimenopausal and postmenopausal women. Your health care provider should do a thorough assessment of your mouth to rule out another cause of the pain, such as thrush or canker sores. The condition usually comes on spontaneously and sometimes it will improve on its own, as well. Unfortunately, there is no specific treatment known to be effective, though the use of benzodiazepines or the anticonvulsant, gabapentin (Neurontin), have helped some women. Estrogen therapy (ET) is not helpful.

ACHES AND PAINS

Headaches   Headaches, especially migraines, are linked to hormones. Migraine headaches usually worsen during perimenopause. This is thought to be related to estrogen withdrawal and erratic hormone levels. Once you reach menopause, headaches improve. Most women whose migraines were menstrual-related will stop having migraines completely.

If you have migraines you need to carefully consider the use of ET. Some women will experience worsening symptoms if they take estrogen. At present there is no way to predetermine which result each woman will have. If you do take ET you should take the lowest effective dose (which you should be doing anyway), and the best choice is one of the nonoral forms that provides a consistent dose, like a transdermal product.

Joint Pain   Joint pain is common in menopause; almost half of postmenopausal women report aching and stiff joints. It occurs more often in women who are overweight or depressed. There is an increase in diagnosis of osteoarthritis in women after menopause, but many women who report joint pain have no evidence of arthritis. Those who already have arthritis often have worsening symptoms after menopause. Treatment after menopause is no different than that used premenopause. Moderate exercise is

What Nurses Know . . .

Nonsteroidal anti-inflammatory drugs (NSAIDs) like ibuprofen (Advil or Motrin) are more effective for musculoskeletal pain than acetaminophen (Tylenol). They not only relieve the pain but also help decrease the inflammation that is causing pain.

NSAIDs can cause gastrointestinal (GI) distress. Always take them with food. If you have a history of stomach ulcers or other stomach problems talk to your health care provider before using NSAIDs. They can make ulcers worse and even cause GI bleeding.

critical for joint health. You really need to keep those joints moving, which strengthens the muscles that support the joint and ensures a good blood flow to supply nutrients and clear away waste products. OTC medications are usually sufficient for pain control when needed. There is no evidence that ET is an effective treatment for joint pain or arthritis in menopausal women.

MENTAL HEALTH

When my mother went through menopause she was a mental case. She was depressed, had anxiety, and was in and out of the hospital. So I was really nervous. But, nothing. Never had any problems.   LIZ

I was a bitch! There was a lot going on in my life at the time, though, and maybe I would have been a bitch anyway. It's hard to say.   SUSAN

Without estrogen I was prone to be pretty depressed. Estrogen keeps me more even.   FRAN

I never had anxiety before menopause. Now, with every hot flash I get an anxiety attack. And every time it feels so real that I have to talk myself through it, "It's the hot flash, you're not about to die, it's the hot flash, nothing horrible is going to happen, it's just the hot flash, oh my god maybe this time it's not ..." KRISTINE

We've all heard the jokes and read the stories about half-crazed menopausal women. There is good news and bad news. First the bad news—going through perimenopause does cause mood swings, irritability, anxiety, depression, memory problems, and difficulty concentrating in many women. The good news—it doesn't last. These symptoms decrease as you transition though perimenopause. And once you hit menopause they usually resolve completely.

Some women are more likely to have problems than others. If you had depression or anxiety before menopause, had PMS with your periods, or feel like you're under a great deal of stress, you are more likely to have mood and behavioral symptoms during the menopausal transition.

Depression We know that the risk of depression is greatest when hormone levels vary, such as during pregnancy, postpartum, or PMS. So it is not surprising that perimenopause causes depression in many women. The encouraging thing is that if you never had depression before perimenopause then it is highly unlikely that you will have it after menopause.

Depression is a real illness. You can't just "snap out of it." Often when we say we're "depressed" it is a transient feeling of frustration, disappointment, or sadness related to a tough situation in our life, and after a few days or so we are able to pick ourselves up and move on. The problem is when you can't pick yourself up, feelings of sadness and hopelessness linger or worsen, causing major disruption in your life. It can affect your job, your relationships, and your physical health. At its worst it can make you feel like you don't want to live anymore. If this happens to you, get help. Counseling and medication can be very effective for even

What Nurses Know...

Symptoms of depression vary from vague feelings of unhappiness that don't go away to constantly crying for no reason. If you have any of the following symptoms for two weeks or more, talk to your provider and look into counseling.

- *Loss of interest in activities*
- *Feeling sad or down*
- *Feeling hopeless or worthless*
- *Crying for no reason*
- *Problems sleeping*
- *Difficulty focusing or concentrating*
- *Difficulty making decisions*
- *Irritability*
- *Restlessness*
- *Unusual fatigue or weakness*
- *Loss of interest in sex*
- *Unintentional weight loss*
- *Unexplained weight gain*
- *Unexplained physical symptoms like back pain, headaches, or no appetite*

If you have any thoughts of hurting yourself, get help immediately. If you find yourself taking chances with your safety—driving dangerously, overmedicating yourself, drinking excessively, and so on—get help immediately.

the worst depression, and in two or three weeks you will be feeling much better.

Anxiety   It is natural to feel anxious in certain situations and, in fact, anxiety can be a good thing. It can prime us to perform at our best. Anxiety is a problem when it is constant or severe and interferes with your ability to function. Anxiety that has no specific cause is called free-floating or generalized anxiety disorder. Stress does not cause generalized anxiety disorder, but it can worsen it.

Women with hot flashes are more likely to report anxiety. It is unclear what the connection is, but it is not thought to be *because* they are having hot flashes. Most of the time the anxiety comes before the hot flashes.

Depression and anxiety often go hand in hand. Effective treatment is available for both. The biggest barrier to getting treatment is the stigma attached. Depression and anxiety symptoms are exactly that—symptoms—and they should be treated as such. There is no shame in taking care of yourself, whether you are seeking treatment for depression or hypertension.

Cognitive Functioning

I don't know…it's been kind of a gradual thing, but I've definitely noticed changes. I'm more forgetful. I just can't keep names and faces straight anymore. And sometimes I just go blank—a brain freeze. Or some of my words don't come out right. I don't know how much of it is years and how much is menopause.   SUSAN

Words will escape me more than they used to. But other than that I really haven't noticed anything. I've been in graduate school since menopause and maybe that helps—my brain is certainly getting a workout! I do find that I can't study intensely for as many hours as I did when I was younger.   KRISTINE

I forget things more now than I ever did. I lose things too. And I have more trouble focusing.   FRAN

If you feel like your memory is shot and you can't keep two coherent thoughts in your head at the same time, don't despair. Thinking processes, also called cognitive functioning, decline during perimenopause but return to normal postmenopause. And your memory is probably not nearly as bad as you think. About 60 percent of women report memory problems during perimenopause. But when women reporting memory loss were given memory tests in studies, there was no evidence of memory problems unless they were depressed; depression can cause problems with memory and concentration. Stress and overall physical health also have an effect on memory changes during the menopausal transition. Managing stress and staying healthy and active can help keep you focused and mentally sharp through this time.

Treatment

EXERCISE

Exercise has many benefits beyond physical fitness and cardiovascular health. Studies show that 30 minutes of exercise a day can make a big improvement in mood and lessen depression and anxiety symptoms. It also improves cognitive functioning and lowers your risk of dementia as you get older. Exercise increases your self-esteem, relaxes tense muscles, distracts you from focusing on problems, raises endorphin levels in your blood, and lowers levels of the stress hormone, cortisol.

COUNSELING

Counseling can be very helpful if you are having difficulty adjusting to the changes in your life during this time, or if you are experiencing new onset of anxiety and depression or worsening of prior symptoms. Finding the right counselor is essential. Start by asking your health care provider for recommendations. Talk to friends and family members; you'll be surprised how many people are getting therapy today. Find a counseling center in your area and contact them for information on local therapists.

Check out the credentials of anyone you are considering going to. Ask them about their training and experience, including what certifications they have, how long they've been in practice, and whether they have experience treating clients with problems similar to yours.

Give yourself a little time to find the right person. Don't settle on the first counselor you see. Plan on making a number of phone calls and a few visits to different counselors before deciding. It's not unusual to feel nervous with someone at first, but after that, if you don't feel like you can talk easily and safely about what is bothering you the most, you need to find a different counselor. Therapy with the wrong counselor is not only ineffective; it can be harmful.

Many therapists who provide counseling cannot prescribe medications. They will consult with your primary care provider

What Nurses Know . . .

Money Matters

Check your health insurance policy before your first appointment. Most policies cover counseling services but there may be specific steps you must take in order to get visits paid for. Some policies require you to notify the health insurance company before you start, or will only cover services if you see certain therapists.

If you don't have health insurance, ask the therapist if they offer a sliding fee scale. Check around before seeing someone who doesn't offer this; there is certain to be a clinic or individual therapist in your area who does.

What Nurses Know ...

Finding the right counselor is essential. Therapy with the wrong counselor is not only ineffective; it can be harmful. After the first couple of visits ask yourself these questions:

Do I trust this person?

Do I have a good rapport with this person?

Did I feel like this person was judging me in anyway?

Do I feel like they "get it"?

How do I feel as the time for the visit nears?

How do I feel when I leave?

If any answers are unsatisfactory—find another counselor.

if medications are needed. If your therapist does prescribe medications make sure they consult with your primary care provider and that everyone has an updated list of the medications you're on.

COMPLEMENTARY AND ALTERNATIVE MEDICINE

There are a number of complementary and alternative therapies that are used to treat depression and anxiety. Many people find them helpful, though there is little scientific evidence to support their use. You must be as careful in choosing a complementary and alternative medicine (CAM) treatment as choosing traditional treatments. This is especially true of supplements and herbal medicine, which can have bad side effects or may interact with other drugs you are taking.

Some safe CAM therapies you may want to give a try:

- *Acupuncture* has been found to be helpful in the treatment of depression and anxiety. For further information on acupuncture see the discussion in Chapter 3, Hot Flashes and Night Sweats.

- *Aromatherapy* uses concentrated essential oils. They can be applied directly to the skin, used in the bath, or diffused into the air. Aromatherapy is relaxing and can be helpful in relieving stress and lessening anxiety. It may help improve your mood but is *not* effective for moderate or severe depression.

- *Light Therapy* uses prolonged exposure to bright light of a certain wavelength to relieve depression. It is very effective for winter depression, also known as seasonal affective disorder, and recent studies suggests that it may be helpful for other depression, as well.

- *Relaxation Techniques* include meditation, guided imagery, and progressive muscle relaxation. They are used to create a state of calm focus and relaxation. Yoga and tai chi are also relaxation approaches that many women have used successfully.

- *Music Therapy* has been shown to be very effective at relieving stress, anxiety, and depression. The type of music depends on you and what you enjoy, though soothing sounds are usually best if you are stressed or anxious.

HERBS

There are a number of different herbs that have been found to be helpful in relieving symptoms of depression and anxiety during the menopausal years. Studies show that St. John's Wort is very effective at treating mild-to-moderate depression. Some studies show that it is as effective as selective serotonin reuptake inhibitors (SSRIs), the most commonly prescribed antidepressant medications. St. John's Wort is relatively safe; the most common side effects are stomach upset, rash, headache, and dizziness.

Black cohosh has been shown to be helpful with mood changes, as well. Ginseng has shown some promise but more research is needed before it can be recommended. Neither gingko nor valerian appears to be helpful at all.

What Nurses Know...

DO NOT take any product containing kava if you have any of the following:

- History of alcohol abuse
- History of liver problems
- History of kidney problems
- A bleeding disorder
- Within two weeks of any surgery

If you are taking kava and have any of the following, report it to your provider right away:

- Yellowing skin (jaundice)
- Unusual fatigue
- Abdominal pain
- Loss of appetite
- Nausea or vomiting
- Joint pain

Kava has been shown to relieve anxiety and improve mood, but you have to be very careful with it. It has been shown to cause severe liver disease, including liver failure. In fact, some countries, including the United Kingdom, have banned its use altogether. In the United States the Food and Drug Administration has issued an advisory stating that anyone with liver disease should contact their physician before taking any product that contains kava.

Alert

DO NOT use kava, St. John's Wort, or valerian with other antidepressant or antianxiety medications. It can lead to a dangerous overdose.
Kava, St. John's Wort, and valerian interact with a number of other medications as well, so be sure to check with your provider before taking them.

You should always talk with your provider before starting any herb or supplement. They can interact with numerous other medications.

You should not try to treat depression by yourself. It is important to have a professional involved who can help you through it and monitor your progress.

MEDICATIONS

Medication can be very helpful if you are struggling with depression and anxiety and other measures have not helped. The most

What Nurses Know . . .

There are many different SSRIs and SNRIs out there, and sometimes it takes trial and error to find the right one and the right dose for you. If one doesn't work or the side effects bother you, try a different one. Or ask about starting at a lower dose and slowly increasing it as your body adjusts to the medication.

Don't give up on the first try. When used correctly, SSRIs and SNRIs can really make a difference. They should not, however, have you walking around in la-la land.

commonly used antidepressants are either medications called SSRIs (selective serotonin reuptake inhibitors) or SNRIs (serotonin and norepinephrine reuptake inhibitors). SSRIs and SNRIs are medications that act on chemicals in the brain to relieve depression and anxiety. They are not habit-forming. It usually takes at least two to three weeks to feel better once you start taking them, though some people report feeling better much earlier.

The most commonly prescribed antianxiety medications are the SSRIs and SNRIs, benzodiazepines, or a drug called buspirone. Benzodiazepines are the medications that are commonly known as sedatives. Whereas SSRIs need time to build up to a certain level and then control symptoms by maintaining that steady level, benzodiazepines work immediately and are used on an "as-needed" basis. They are habit-forming, though, and you can build up a tolerance over time. So they generally should not be used daily or for extended periods of time. Buspirone is an antianxiety medication that is often prescribed as an additional drug when SSRIs alone aren't controlling anxiety symptoms.

It is important to find the right drug and the right dosage that works for you. Antidepressant and antianxiety medications are not meant to make you feel like life is wonderful all the time, nor are they meant to make you numb. They are meant to take the edge off the emotional extremes that disrupt and limit your life.

Resources

GENERAL HEALTH

American Cancer Society

For general information about cancer prevention go to the Health Information Seekers link under the heading, "I need information for …"
www.cancer.org

American Heart Association

Offers comprehensive information on cardiovascular health including prevention of stroke and heart attack. The "Healthy

Lifestyle" link has information on how to live a heart-healthy life, and has a section devoted specifically to women.
www.americanheart.org

Medline Plus: Health Screening
This Web site has updated information and resources on recommended health screenings.
www.nlm.nih.gov/medlineplus/healthscreening.html

National Heart, Lung and Blood Institute
This is a branch of the National Institutes for Health. On their Web site, under the "Public" heading, you can find extensive information on cardiovascular health. They also have a section specific to women.
www.nhlbi.nih.gov/index.htm

National Research Center for Women and Families
This site gives you easy-to-understand information on the latest cancer research as well as other topics important to women.
www.center4research.org

MENTAL HEALTH

American Association of Pastoral Counselors
This association supports psychological services that are grounded in theology and spirituality. The Web site has a directory of certified pastoral counselors.
www.aapc.org

American Psychological Association
The Web site for this professional organization offers consumer information on mind/body health, including sections on aging, stress, anxiety, and depression.
www.helping.apa.org

MedlinePlus: Mental Health
Offers comprehensive information on mental health and links to other resources.
www.nlm.nih.gov/medlineplus/mentalhealth.html

Mental Health America
Offers extensive information on mental health that is searchable by audience, disorder, or treatment.
www.nmha.org

National Association of Social Workers
This professional organization's Web site maintains a list of clinical social workers who have met national certification guidelines.
www.naswdc.org

National Mental Health Information Center
Comprehensive information from the U.S. Department of Health and Human Services.
http://mentalhealth.samhsa.gov

Psychology Today
User-friendly site geared to consumers with engaging articles and all kinds of information.
www.psychologytoday.com

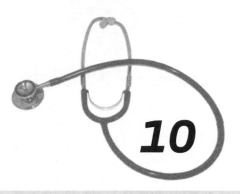

Being Beautiful

The aging of women is a big joke in our society; but I'm not laughing. I feel very alone at times. JOYCE

I'm determined to grow old gracefully. I believe you can really look good no matter how old you are. Though I have to admit, I've noticed my eyes and it does bother me a little. SUSAN

As I approached 50 I began to notice that I was fading into invisibility out in the world. Strange when you no longer register, as if you could just—poof!—disappear, and the people walking by would never even notice. KRISTINE

I find the changes in my body interesting, for one thing. I'm amused by the signs of aging...such as the pronounced smile lines...I remind myself of my Mom, and I like that. CAROLE

There is no way around it; menopause, along with aging, will change your body. Weight control gets even more difficult. You can't find your waist anymore. New wrinkles seem to appear overnight.

That doesn't mean you no longer feel good about your body. You still can have skin that glows and a strong toned body. It starts with good health, physical and mental. You cannot have glowing skin and a strong body without a nutritious diet and regular exercise. You cannot have vitality and grace without a sense of ease and joyfulness with the world.

Feeling good about your body is not about trying to look young. You won't feel good if you're 55 years of age and your goal is to be wrinkle-free and have an hourglass shape. Trying to achieve that will cost you untold time, money, and endless frustration.

You can achieve beauty. Being beautiful has nothing to do with age. It is about strength and grace and healthfulness. It is about how you carry yourself as you move through the world. It is about knowing who you are and having a style that embodies it.

What Nurses Know . . .

Taking care of our skin is not just about looking good. It's about our health. We don't usually think of our skin as an organ, but that is what it is. In fact, our skin is the largest organ of our body. Unwrapped it would cover about 20 square feet and weigh about eight pounds. Our skin has a number of important functions. It protects us against infection, dehydration, harmful chemicals, and keeps all our other organs safe from the wear and tear of exposure to the environment. It is waterproof and helps keep our body temperature regulated. Finally, it is a sensory organ—our brain's contact with the outside world.

Being Beautiful

A BRIEF REVIEW OF THE ANATOMY AND PHYSIOLOGY OF THE SKIN

Your skin has three layers. The outer layer is the epidermis. It is made of tough protein called keratin. There are no blood vessels or nerves in the epidermis. As the old outermost layer of cells (stratum corneum) die and flake off, new cells grow from the inside out to replace them. This process takes about five weeks.

The middle layer is the dermis. It is made of collagen and elastin and gives the skin its elasticity and strength. It contains blood vessels, nerves, hair follicles, and glands. There are two types of glands. Sweat glands help regulate body temperature and get rid of waste by producing sweat. Sebaceous glands produce an oily substance called sebum that lubricates our skin and hair.

The deepest layer is the subcutis, which has a layer of fat. It acts as a cushion and insulation, as well as a source of fuel if we don't eat enough.

Melanin is the pigmented substance that gives our skin color. Its purpose is to protect us from the harmful ultraviolet rays of the sun. The more sun exposure you have, the more melanin your skin produces. That is why people who are indigenous to regions where the sun shines brightest for longer periods of time have darker skin. It is also why sun exposure causes tanning in lighter-skinned people.

SKIN, AGING, AND MENOPAUSE

It's difficult looking at a face that's sagging in places you didn't believe could happen…and, oh, the neck! HOPE

As with many of the changes we undergo as we get older, the ones we see in our skin are a combination of the processes of aging and menopause. There are a number of different things that affect how our skin ages, including basic aging with time, photoaging due to sun exposure, stresses from the environment, and estrogen supply.

Estrogen helps maintain the skin's tone, elasticity, and moisture. It keeps collagen from breaking down, maintains elastic fibers in the dermis, helps the epidermis hold onto its water content, and plays a role in regulating the activity of the sebaceous glands. So when estrogen supply decreases with menopause, our skin becomes thinner, less elastic, and drier. It is estimated that we lose about 30 percent of skin collagen in the first five years after menopause (it slows down after that) and our skin gets one percent thinner every year during the first 15 to 18 years. Atrophy and decreased collagen result in loss of elasticity and tone, which leads to wrinkles. Decreased water and sebaceous secretions means our skin is drier and also less supple.

Currently, estrogen therapy (ET) is not approved to prevent skin aging. With the known risks and lingering uncertainties around estrogen use, it is not recommended that you take it solely for that purpose. There is research that suggests that topical estrogen products (applied directly to the skin) are effective in slowing collagen loss. Some women have been known to use their vaginal estrogen cream on their face. Some claim that it works well, while others complain of headaches and even vaginal bleeding when they use it. Remember, medications applied to the skin are absorbed into your system. If you are applying a product both vaginally and on your face you will be absorbing more than your prescription intends. Talk to your health care provider before devising your own treatment. Also, there is no evidence that over-the-counter (OTC) phytoestrogen creams are effective in preventing or reducing wrinkles. Think twice before spending money on them.

There are some aspects of skin aging you have no control over. Genetics is one of them. Take a look at your parents' skin and you will probably see a good predictor of how your skin will age. However, keep in mind that your parents' generation went through young adulthood before we knew about the ravages of the sun and the dangers of cigarettes. So they may have had exposures that worsened their skin's aging that you haven't had.

There are things that you can do to minimize wrinkling as you get older. Stay out of the sun, and if you smoke, quit. Sun exposure causes most of the damage to your skin over time, not aging or the loss of estrogen. And smoking makes it much, much worse.

Staying out of the sun is the best thing you can do for your skin. Skin changes related to basic aging with time include a loss of collagen and elasticity in the dermis. This causes fine wrinkles and slight sagginess. Most of the rest of the changes you see are due to the sun. If you're not convinced of the amount of damage the sun does, just compare the skin on your face and the back of your hands with that on an area of your body that hasn't been exposed to the sun, such as the lower part of your breasts.

Use sunscreen everyday. An easy way to remember is to use one of the many moisturizers that have sunscreen in them. Wear a hat when you'll be outside for a while and wear sunglasses to prevent squinting.

If you smoke, quit. Smoking accelerates skin aging. Not only will smokers start wrinkling earlier than nonsmokers, the damage to their skin will be worse. Studies have found that smokers have more than two and a half times as many wrinkles as nonsmokers, and ET does not help. The repeated puckering of the mouth as a smoker inhales on a cigarette, and the constant squinting against the cigarette smoke result in "smoker's face," characterized by deep wrinkles around the mouth and eyes.

Exposure to harsh environments will damage your skin, as well. Protect your skin from extremes of heat and cold. Wear scarves and use a good moisturizer in winter weather. Stay well-hydrated and take the precautions with sun exposure outlined above during the summer.

Skin care starts from the inside out. Good nutrition and plenty of water are essential for healthy skin. All the moisturizers in the world won't help you if you're not drinking enough water. Foods high in antioxidants help control skin cell damage caused by free radicals. Look for foods that are high in vitamins C and E. Blueberries are one of the best food sources of antioxidants.

HAIR, AGING, AND MENOPAUSE

We expect our hair to get gray as we get older. However, many women are not prepared for other hair changes that menopause may bring. As estrogen levels decline, the ratio between estrogen and androgen shifts. Some women find they have more hair on their face and less hair on their head.

About half of postmenopausal women will notice thinning of the hair on their head. If you have significant hair loss (alopecia), talk to your health care provider about treatment. There are two prescription medications available to treat alopecia: minoxidil and finasteride. You and your health care provider can decide if you would benefit from their use.

There are a great many products out there being touted as treatments for hair loss, but there is no evidence to support those claims. Do not be taken in by the advertisements. A number of OTC hair products will make your hair *appear* thicker and fuller, but other than the two medications mentioned earlier, there are no products that actually increase hair growth or stop hair loss.

• •

Hair Loss Myths

The following are some of the false claims used to promote hair products:

- Increasing blood flow to the scalp will stop hair loss and increase hair growth
- You can increase the number of hair follicles on your scalp, thereby increasing hair growth
- Special hair products will not damage your hair and cause hair loss, while others will
- Certain herbal products, vitamins, or natural supplements will stop hair loss or promote hair growth
- Unplugging hair follicles will promote hair growth.

Again, there are products that will make your hair appear healthier and thicker, but they will NOT stop hair loss or promote hair growth.

Hair Care and Products   Even if you don't have a problem with hair loss after menopause, you will notice that your hair has become thinner and more brittle. Your hair care routine can make a big difference in your hair's appearance. Certain hair care routines, like frequent blow drying, bleaching, tight braiding, hot curlers, or flat irons, can further damage your hair, resulting in thinner hair coverage. Some experts recommend that women with thinning hair wash their hair with a gentle shampoo every day. Hair will look fuller if it isn't weighed down by the buildup of dirt and oils. There are also hair products available that make hair look thicker by roughening the hair cuticle. Hair color and perms will have this effect, as well, but be careful not to overuse them and end up damaging your hair.

Hirsutism   Hirsutism is excessive hair growth in women that manifests in a male distribution pattern. Hirsutism brought on by menopause is usually mild. Women notice an overall fuzzy hair growth on their face, or a few long stray hairs on their chin. Most of the time it is easily managed with mechanical measures such as plucking, bleaching, shaving, electrolysis, and laser treatments. There is a prescription cream available, Vaniqua, that treats unwanted facial hair. It works by slowing the growth and decreasing the size of the hair. It helps about 60 percent of women who use it, and about half of those have a marked improvement. The change is not permanent; once you stop using it, hair growth returns to its preuse condition.

What Nurses Know...

Stat Fact

Hirsutism affects about eight percent of women in the United States—over four million women.

BODY CHANGES

What about the men-o-pot?! You know, that pouch under the belly button that gets a permanent wrinkle underneath from your skin holding it up? Just try to get rid of it ... ha ha!   FRAN

I never gained any weight, but my jeans fit differently. I'm still in the same size, but some of my jeans—there's no way I can get them past my hips!   SUSAN

Where'd my waist go? I really miss it!   KRISTINE

After menopause your body shape changes. You are much more likely to be shaped like an apple than a pear. Even if you don't gain any weight, your body fat gets redistributed around your middle.

Women tend to gain an average of six pounds in the years after menopause. This might not sound like a lot, but it is enough to affect your health, especially if you are among the majority of women who are overweight to begin with. And when fat is concentrated around the abdomen, as happens with menopause, you are at greater risk for heart disease than if it is more evenly distributed throughout your body.

Preventing weight gain is key; we all know how difficult it is to take weight off and keep it off. Following is weight control advice

What Nurses Know...

Because something works in a study doesn't guarantee it's going to work for you in your real life, and vice versa.

*If your weight control plan is to succeed, it has to fit **your lifestyle**, it has to build on **your strengths**, it has to overcome **your weaknesses**.*

based on the latest research. Use these strategies as guidelines, talk to your health care provider, and keep trying.

WEIGHT CONTROL STRATEGIES

I joined Weight Watchers to keep my weight under control and it worked. I joined a gym this year too, plus exercise helps keep me centered.   CAROLE

I've been a runner for a long time. It used to be if my weight went up I'd just increase my mileage for a few weeks and away it would go. Not so easy anymore! But I still always feel so much better when I run regularly, and it definitely helps me control my weight.   KRISTINE

When talking about weight we need to be talking about *controlling* weight. As hard as losing weight may be, the real challenge is keeping it off. In weight-loss studies there are four strategies that are consistently associated with successful long-term weight control:

Eating a low-calorie, low-fat diet. There are all kinds of diets based on lowering caloric intake, eliminating certain foods, or eating a calculated combination of carbohydrates, protein, and fats. Studies have mixed results about what combination of carbohydrates, protein, and fats are best for weight loss, but they all agree on one thing: **It is the decrease in calories, not the diet composition, that leads to weight loss in all of them.**

The diet that most often comes out on top, though, is a low-calorie, low-fat diet. To lose weight you should eat about 1,200 to 1,500 calories a day with no more than 30 percent of them coming from fat. Once you're at your ideal body weight you can increase your calories to a level that allows you to maintain your weight while still keeping your fat intake at 30 percent. You can find calorie calculators online that help you figure out what your daily calorie needs are. Make sure you use one from a reliable source, like MayoClinic.com or WebMD.

After menopause it is important to make sure you eat enough protein, especially if you are dieting. As we get older we lose

What Nurses Know...

When it comes to weight loss, it is **how much** you eat that matters. However, when it comes to health, **what** you eat is just as important.

lean body mass, and dieting increases that loss. Lean body mass is everything that isn't fat, including muscle. Eating higher amounts of dietary proteins, while still keeping your overall calorie count down, will help you preserve your lean body mass. Vegetable proteins are better than animal proteins (meat); they have a positive effect on cholesterol levels and have been shown to lower blood pressure in people with high blood pressure. This type of diet has a much higher fiber content, as well.

Eating regular meals. Eating regular meals spaced throughout the day has been shown to increase weight loss, starting with breakfast. People who regularly eat breakfast are more likely to maintain their weight loss than people who don't.

Maintaining a consistent diet seven days a week, 365 days a year. Some people think that giving themselves permission to eat treats on weekends or holidays will relieve food cravings and help them stay on track over the long term. Studies repeatedly show that women who consistently stayed with healthy eating habits lost more weight and kept it off for longer periods of time than women who didn't. This doesn't mean you can't indulge in the occasional treat, and in fact, allowing some flexibility in your diet has been linked with long-term success. No one can maintain rigid self-denial forever, and those who try are more likely to sooner or later lose complete control and overeat.

Frequent self-monitoring of body weight and food intake. Checking your weight on a regular basis and keeping records of food intake promotes long-term success in weight control. When you keep a record of what you eat, how much you eat, and when you eat it, you pay attention to your food intake and the decisions you make about food.

In addition to these four strategies, a number of others are also associated with successful weight control.

High levels of physical activity. Recent research shows that engaging in high levels of physical activity won't necessarily

• •

How Intense Is Moderate Intensity?

How do you tell the intensity level of your exercise? One way is to check your heart rate. For moderate intensity, aim for a heart rate that is 50 to 70 percent of your maximum heart rate, using the following calculation:

- Subtract your age from 220 to get your maximum heart rate (in beats per minute)
- Multiply that number by 0.5 to get the lower limit and by 0.7 for the upper limit
- The result is the range you want your heart rate to be in during moderate-intensity exercise
- Example—You're 50 years of age with a resting heart rate of 70

  - Subtract 50 from 220 for a maximum heart rate of 170 beats per minute
  - Multiply 170 by 0.5 for a lower range of 85 and by 0.7 for an upper range of 117

There are a couple of other ways that also work and don't require all the calculations and trying to take your own pulse while you are exercising.

- If you're a walker, get a pedometer. One hundred steps a minute represents a moderate level of intensity, so aim for 1,500 steps in 15 minutes.
- If you can easily carry on a conversation during the activity, your exercise intensity level is low. If you can carry on a conversation but not easily, your exercise intensity is moderate. If you can't carry on a conversation because you're too out of breath to speak, your exercise intensity is vigorous (too high, unless you're an athlete or exceptionally fit).

So aim for that talking-with-difficulty stride.
Remember—if you haven't been exercising, start off slowly and build up your intensity level and duration over time.

increase weight loss, but it is essential for keeping it off. According to a 2010 study of over 35,000 middle-aged and older women, the only ones who didn't gain weight after menopause were those who averaged an hour of moderate-intensity exercise a day.

Studies that look at the strategies used by people who have successfully lost weight and maintained their weight loss have found that almost all of them have used a combination of dieting and increased activity.

Support. There is strong evidence that the support of family and friends enhances long-term weight control. Results on spousal and partner support is not so straightforward: Sometimes it helps, sometimes it makes no difference, and in some studies partners actually were a bad influence. When a couple is trying to lose weight together, the mutual support is very helpful.

Ongoing support from professionals, such as nutritionists, therapists, or your health care provider, is also effective in maintaining weight loss. Having regular in-person meetings, even if they are as infrequent as every two months, results in greater weight loss and an increased likelihood that you'll keep it off. Phone contact is also helpful, though not as much as in-person support. Some early studies showed that Internet support programs were helpful, but more recent studies found that they are not helpful for the long term. Having that "real" person contact seems to be the key in support programs.

Many people use commercial and professional weight-loss programs and do very well with them. Currently, Weight Watchers is the only program that has been studied, and the research shows it to be successful. Most people state that it is the weekly meetings that make a difference. Having to show up and answer to a group of fellow weight losers for what you ate all week and any changes in your weight helps many people stay on track.

Prevent small gains from becoming big ones. If you do slip back to bad eating habits and start gaining weight, the less you allow yourself to regain the less likely you'll go into a full relapse. It's not the small slipups that do you in; it's letting a slipup become your eating habits again. If you're in perimenopause, now is the time to change your eating and exercise habits, before you start gaining.

WHAT ABOUT WEIGHT-LOSS DRUGS?

Drugs do not have a big place in weight control strategies for a number of reasons. First, any drug carries the risk of side effects, and second, their benefits are limited. Their effect only lasts as long as you are taking the drug and usually you will gain back the weight when the drug is stopped. You cannot stay on weight-loss drugs forever. They have only been tested for safety when used for up to two years. They usually lose their effectiveness after about 6 months of use anyway.

That said, there are situations in which weight-loss drugs can be helpful, primarily if your body mass index is greater than 27 and you have been unsuccessful in prior attempts to lose weight. These drugs should always be used in combination with weight-loss counseling that includes diet changes and exercise. Your plan should be to use the drug to get your weight loss started while you make lifestyle changes that will enhance your chances of long-term success.

The two most commonly used weight-loss drugs approved by the FDA are sibutramine (Meridia) and orlistat (Xenical and Alli). Both have significant side effects.

Sibutramine is a prescription medication. It can increase your heart rate, raise your blood pressure, and cause an irregular heartbeat. It was taken off the market in Europe in 2009 because

What Nurses Know...

Avoid OTC appetite suppressants and weight-loss aids. There is no evidence that they work and many are actually dangerous.

What Nurses Know...

Always read food labels—there are some real surprises out there. The marketing of certain foods can lead to a...let's say misunderstanding, of their health benefits! Along with calorie counts, compare fiber, sugar, carbohydrates, fats (all kinds), protein, and sodium content, as well as vitamin and mineral values. Make sure you look at the serving size. They're not all the same and it makes a big difference in actual values.

it increased the risk of heart attacks, stroke, and other cardiovascular problems in people with certain health problems. It is still approved for use in the United States but the FDA has required the drug's manufacturer to put stronger warnings on the drug label.

Orlistat is available in both prescription strength (Xenical) and OTC strength (Alli). It works by decreasing the body's absorption of fat in the gastrointestinal tract. It frequently will lower cholesterol, as well. Unfortunately, it's not without a price. Fat that isn't being absorbed by your body has to be eliminated. This causes oily stools, urgent need to move your bowels that can result in incontinence, intestinal gas with discharge, abdominal pain, and diarrhea. Many people quit taking orlistat because of these embarrassing side effects. Orlistat also decreases absorption of fat-soluble vitamins, so you need to take a vitamin supplement when you are on it. The FDA recently reported that it is looking into reports of liver damage in people taking orlistat, but they have not recommended any changes in its use.

EXERCISE

As noted earlier, a high level of physical activity is essential for weight control, especially after menopause. Weight control is

● ●

2010 American Heart Association Exercise Recommendations for Healthy Adults

● Everyone needs to engage in moderate-intensity exercise for at least 30 minutes, five days a week, or vigorous-intensity exercise for at least 20 minutes, three days a week.
● A combination of the moderate- and vigorous-intensity exercise can be done to meet the requirement.
● The moderate-intensity requirement of 30 minutes can be done in three episodes of 10 minutes.
● Everyone should engage in muscle strengthening and endurance building activities at least twice a week.

only one of many benefits that exercise offers postmenopausal women. It promotes cardiovascular health, maintains healthy bones, improves strength and balance, and contributes to a sense of well-being.

Getting started is the hardest part. Once you establish a regular routine of exercise the improvements in how you feel will carry you along. The key is making it a priority appointment in your day. There is always a good excuse not to exercise—it's raining outside, you need to spend that hour getting work done, company's coming—whatever it is, it is still just an excuse. You choose how you spend your time in each waking moment. Choose to devote an hour a day to exercise. It will benefit every other aspect of your life.

You should always talk to your health care provider before starting any exercise program. Start slow and gradually build up intensity and duration to prevent injuries. It will also help to prevent frustrations and sore muscles that can undermine your efforts. Find an exercise partner. A brisk walk with a friend gets you in shape and has the added benefit of talk time. Try different types of exercise classes. Walk or ride a bike instead of driving or taking the bus. Set a goal for yourself, a 5K run to participate in, or another activity you currently don't have the strength or endurance to complete. Make sure your goals are realistic. You want a reward at the end, not a reason to beat yourself up. For more information on exercise, see Chapter 6, Bone Health.

Resources

American Academy of Dermatology
You will find information on Aging/Mature Skin if you go to Public, then Conditions/Diseases, then Dermatology A-Z. This site can also help you locate a reputable dermatologist in your area.
www.aad.org/Public/index.html

American Dietetic Association
This public information center on this site offers comprehensive information about nutrition, diet, and weight control, among other things.
www.eatright.org/cps/rde/xchg/ada/hs.xsl/index.html

American Hair Loss Association
This organization works to improve the lives of people affected by hair loss. This Web site has extensive information about hair loss, including a section specifically for women.
www.americanhairloss.org/

CDC: Healthy Weight
This CDC Web site on weight control offers a broad range of information on reaching and maintaining a healthy weight.
www.cdc.gov/healthyweight/index.html

FDA: Make Your Calories Count
An interactive site to learn how to plan a healthy diet and manage your calorie intake.
www.fda.gov/Food/LabelingNutrition/ConsumerInformation/ucm114022.htm

Nutrition.gov
This Web site offers access to all the food and nutrition information the federal government has, including food ingredients and weight management.
www.nutrition.gov

Shape Up America!
The Web site of this nonprofit organization has all kinds of information on healthy weight management, covering diet, exercise, and behavior.
www.shapeup.org/

USDA: The National Agricultural Library
This site lists different government-related Web sites dealing with nutrition, exercise, and food-related health information.
fnic.nal.usda.gov/nal_display/index. php?tax_level=1&info_center=4

Weight Watchers
You don't have to be a member of Weight Watchers to access many of this Web site's features, including extensive information on weight management, helpful tips on things like food shopping and eating out, and healthy cooking ideas.
www.weightwatchers.com/index.aspx

Glossary

Note: Definitions listed here are for use of the word in the context of menopause. Some of the words may have additional meanings in other contexts. For complete definitions refer to a general or medical dictionary.

Acupuncture–a traditional Chinese medicine technique that uses needles for therapeutic purposes.

Amenorrhea–absence of menstrual cycles.

Androgen–sex hormone that is responsible for male characteristics and reproductive activity in males, and plays a role in estrogen production, bone health, and sexual desire in females.

Anovulation–absence of ovulation.

Atherosclerosis–localized lipid-containing plaque in the walls of blood vessels.

Atrophy–decrease in size, wasting.

Biomedical—relating to both biology and medicine.

BMI—body mass index. Indicator of body fat level based on a calculation of the relationship between a person's height and weight.

Calcification—calcium deposits.

Cerebrovascular—pertaining to the blood vessels in the brain.

Climacteric—the period of time from perimenopause to early postmenopause; the transition from premenopause to postmenopause.

Collagen—the main protein present in connective tissue; supports and strengthens skin, bone, and muscle.

Corpus luteum—temporary component of an ovary that develops from the follicle after ovulation. Secretes estrogen and progesterone. Important in proliferation and shedding of endometrium during menstrual cycle.

Cutaneous—pertaining to the skin; includes hair.

Dementia—the deterioration of mental functioning.

Dermis—the middle elastic layer of the skin.

Diuretic—drug or natural substance that increases the output of urine.

Dyspareunia—painful sexual intercourse.

Endocrine—of or relating to the glands that secrete hormones.

Endocrinologist—physician who specializes in hormonal conditions, including menopause, diabetes, and thyroid disease.

Endogenous—originating within the body.

Endometrium—lining of the uterus. Proliferates and then sheds cyclically under the influence of hormones (menstrual cycle).

Epidermis—the outermost layer of the skin.

Etiology—cause of a disease, condition, or syndrome.

Exogenous–originating from outside the body.

Fibrosis–the abnormal growth of fibrous tissue.

First-degree relative–your parents, siblings, and children.

Follicle-stimulating hormone–a hormone secreted by the pituitary gland, which stimulates maturation of ovarian follicles.

Follicular atresia–natural process whereby follicles are broken down and reabsorbed by the body.

Hirsutism–excessive growth of coarse hair in women, manifesting in a male distribution pattern.

Hormone–substance produced by an organ or gland that then travels to another part of the body where it triggers a specific action.

Hyperplasia–the overgrowth of tissue.

Hypertension–high blood pressure. Usually defined as systolic (top number) equal to or greater than 140 and diastolic (lower number) equal to or greater than 90.

Idiopathic–disease, condition, or disorder that has no known cause.

Inhibin B–a hormone secreted by developing follicles that inhibits secretion of FSH by the pituitary gland.

Introitus–the entrance or opening of the vagina.

Lipids–fat substances in the blood; cholesterol, triglycerides.

Luteinizing hormone–a hormone secreted by the pituitary gland that plays a role in maturation of ovarian follicles and triggers ovulation.

Macronutrients–carbohydrate, protein, and fat; nutrients that the body uses in large quantities.

Malaise–generalized feeling of discomfort or feeling unwell.

Melanin–substance that gives skin its color.

Melatonin—hormone involved in regulating sleep and wake cycles.

Menopause—the permanent end of menstruation and reproductive ability.

Metabolic—pertaining to the chemical activity in the body.

Neurotransmitters—chemicals released by one nerve cell that carry a message to another nerve or part of the body.

Oligo-ovulation—infrequent ovulation.

Oligomenorrhea—infrequent menstrual cycles, usually defined as nine or fewer a year.

Osteoclast—cell that breaks down bone tissue.

Osteomalacia—softening of the bones due to deficiency of vitamin D, calcium, and phosphorous.

Osteopenia—condition of low bone density, though not as low as seen in osteoporosis.

Osteoporosis—condition of weak, porous bones due to low bone density that puts the individual at risk for fractures.

Ovulation—the release of an ovum (egg) from a mature ovarian follicle.

Pathological—due to disease, diseased.

Perimenopause—the period of transition from reproductive years to menopause.

Phytoestrogen—hormone-like substances found in plants.

Placebo—a "fake" pill or treatment used in research.

Premenopause—the years preceding menopause.

Progesterone—hormone produced by the ovary that is involved in regulation of the menstrual cycle, development of the placenta during pregnancy, and lactation.

Pulmonary embolism—a blood clot in the blood vessels of the lungs.

Stratum corneum–the layer of dead skin cells on the outer surface of the epidermis.

Thrombosis–a blood clot that forms in a blood vessel (if breaks off and travels through bloodstream, it is an embolus).

Topical–applied to the skin or mucous membranes.

Transdermal–absorbed through the skin.

Vasomotor–motor activity of blood vessels, includes constriction and dilation.

Vertebral–having to do with the vertebrae (individual bones of the spinal column).

Bibliography

Chapter 1

Amundsen, D. W., & Diers, C. J. (1970). The age of menopause in classical Greece and Rome. *Human Biology; an International Record of Research, 42*(1), 79-86.

Amundsen, D. W., & Diers, C. J. (1973). The age of menopause in Medieval Europe. *Human Biology; an International Record of Research, 45*(4), 605-612.

Banks, E. (2002). From dogs' testicles to mares' urine: The origins and contemporary use of hormonal therapy for the menopause. *Feminist Review, 72*, 2-25.

Burger, H. G. (1996). The menopausal transition. *Baillière's Clinical Obstetrics and Gynaecology, 10*(3), 347-359.

Caillouette, J. C., & Sharp, C. F. (1997). Vaginal pH as a marker for bacterial pathogens and menopausal status. *American Journal of Obstetrics and Gynecology, 176*(6), 1270-1277.

CDC. (2004). *United States Life Tables. National Vital Statistics Reports.* Retrieved March 3, 2010, from http://cdc.gov/nchs/data/nvsr/nvsr56/nvsr56_09.pdf

De Bruin, J. P., Bovenhuis, H., Van Noord, P. A. H., Pearson, P. L., Van Arendonk, J. A. M., Te Velde, E. R., et al. (2001). The role of genetic factors in age at natural menopause. *Human Reproduction, 16*(9), 2014-2018.

Fogel, C. I., & Woods, N. F. (2008). *Women's health care in advanced practice nursing.* New York: Springer Publishing Company.

Grady, D. (2006). Management of menopausal symptoms. *The New England Journal of Medicine, 355*(22), 2338-2347.

Houck, J. A. (2006). *Hot and bothered: Women, medicine, and menopause in modern America.* Cambridge, MA: Harvard University Press.

McCrea, F. B. (1983). The politics of menopause: The "discovery" of a deficiency disease. *Social Problems, 31*(1), 111-123.

McKinlay, S. M., Brambilla, D. J., & Posner, J. G. (2008). "Reprint of" the normal menopause transition. *Maturitas, 61*(1-2), 4-16.

Menopause The Musical. Retrieved March 7, 2010, from http://www.menopausethemusical.com/

Neugarten, B. L., Wood, V., Kraines, R. J., & Loomis, B. (1964). Women's attitudes toward the menopause. *Obstetrical & Gynecological Survey, 19*(1), 149-151.

Soules, M. R., Sherman, S., Parrott, E., Rebar, R., Santoro, N., Utian, W., et al. (2001a). Executive summary: Stages of Reproductive Aging Workshop (STRAW). *Climacteric, 4*(4), 267-272.

Soules, M. R., Sherman, S., Parrott, E., Rebar, R., Santoro, N., Utian, W., et al. (2001b). Stages of Reproductive Aging Workshop (STRAW). *Journal of Women's Health & Gender-Based Medicine, 10*(9), 843-848.

Swartzman, L. C., & Leiblum, S. R. (1987). Changing perspectives on the menopause. *Journal of Psychosomatic Obstetrics & Gynecology, 6*(1), 11-24.

Tilt, E. J. (1882). *The change of life in health and disease: Diseases of the ganglionic nervous system incidental to women at the decline of life.* Philadelphia: P. Blaksiston, Son & Co. Retrieved December 11, 2009, from http://books. google.com/books?id=5aI9bnek-30C&printsec=frontcover&d q=tilt+edward+the+change+of+life&source=bl&ots=jr5RNkp7 J4&sig=9c5xv95aNKajW2T8ajeokl7oHMc&hl=en&ei=MTeRS_ K9DNDU8Abz2Mj2BA&sa=X&oi=book_result&ct=result&resn um=1&ved=0CAYQ6AEwAA#v=onepage&q=&f=false

Utian, W. H. (1997). Menopause—A modern perspective from a controversial history. *Maturitas, 26*(2), 73-82.

van Asselt, K. M., Kok, H. S., Pearson, P. L., Dubas, J. S., Peeters, P. H. M., Te Velde, E. R., et al. (2004). Heritability of menopausal age in mothers and daughters. *Fertility and Sterility, 82*(5), 1348-1351.

Wilson, R. A., & Wilson, T. A. (1963). The fate of the nontreated postmenopausal woman: A plea for the maintenance of adequate estrogen from puberty to the grave. *Journal of the American Geriatrics Society, 11*, 347-362.

Woods, N. F., Mitchell, E. S., Percival, D. B., & Smith-DiJulio, K. (2009). Is the menopausal transition stressful? Observations of perceived stress from the Seattle Midlife Women's Health Study. *Menopause, 16*(1), 90-97.

Chapter 2

Burger, H. G. (1996). The menopausal transition. *Baillière's Clinical Obstetrics and Gynaecology, 10*(3), 347-359.

Burger, H. G., Dudley, E. C., Robertson, D. M., & Dennerstein, L. (2002). Hormonal changes in the menopause transition. *Recent Progress in Hormone Research, 57*(1), 257-275.

Burger, H. G., Hale, G. E., Robertson, D. M., & Dennerstein, L. (2007). A review of hormonal changes during the menopausal transition: Focus on findings from the Melbourne Women's Midlife Health Project. *Human Reproduction Update, 13*(6), 559-565.

CDC. (2008). *Hysterectomy in the United States, 2000-2004.* Retrieved March 3, 2010, from http://www.cdc.gov/reproductivehealth/WomensRH/00-04-FS_Hysterectomy.htm

Davison, S. L., Bell, R., Donath, S., Montalto, J. G., & Davis, S. R. (2005). Androgen levels in adult females: Changes with age, menopause, and oophorectomy. *Journal of Clinical Endocrinology & Metabolism, 90*(7), 3847-3853.

De Bruin, M. L., Huisbrink, J., Hauptmann, M., Kuenen, M. A., Ouwens, G. M., van't Veer, M. B., et al. (2008). Treatment-related risk factors for premature menopause following Hodgkin lymphoma. *Blood, 111*(1), 101-108.

Goodwin, P. J., Ennis, M., Pritchard, K. I., Trudeau, M., & Hood, N. (1999). Risk of menopause during the first year after breast cancer diagnosis. *Journal of Clinical Oncology, 17*(8), 2365-2370.

Grady, D. (2006). Management of menopausal symptoms. *The New England Journal of Medicine, 355*(22), 2338-2347.

Gruber, C. J., Tschugguel, W., Schneeberger, C., & Huber, J. C. (2002). Production and actions of estrogens. *The New England Journal of Medicine, 346*(5), 340-352.

Houck, J. A. (2002). How to treat a menopausal woman: A history, 1900 to 2000. *Current Woman's Health Reports, 2*(5), 349-355.

Kurjak, A., & Kupesic, S. (1995). Ovarian senescence and its significance on uterine and ovarian perfusion. *Fertility and Sterility, 64*(3), 532-537.

McKinlay, S. M., Brambilla, D. J., & Posner, J. G. (2008). "Reprint of" the normal menopause transition. *Maturitas, 61*(1-2), 4-16.

MMWR. (2002). *Hysterectomy Surveillance—United States, 1994-1999.* Retrieved March 3, 2010, from http://www.cdc.gov/mmwr/preview/mmwrhtml/ss5105a1.htm

Shifren, L. (2005). The role of testosterone therapy in postmenopausal women: Position statement of the North American Menopause Society [NAMS position statement]. *Menopause, 12*(5), 497-511.

Shoupe, D., Parker, W. H., Broder, M. S., Liu, Z., Farquhar, C., & Berek, J. S. (2007). Elective oophorectomy for benign gynecological disorders. *Menopause, 14*(3), 580-585.

Sklar, C. (2005). Maintenance of ovarian function and risk of premature menopause related to cancer treatment. *JNCI Cancer Spectrum,* 25-27.

Soules, M. R., Sherman, S., Parrott, E., Rebar, R., Santoro, N., Utian, W., et al. (2001). Executive summary: Stages of reproductive aging workshop (STRAW). *Climacteric, 4*(4), 267-272.

Tarcan, T., Park, K., Goldstein, I., Maio, G., Fassina, A., Krane, R. J., et al. (1999). Histomorphometric analysis of age-related structural changes in human clitoral cavernosal tissue. *The Journal of Urology, 161*(3), 940-944.

Chapter 3

Borud, E. K., Alraek, T., White, A., & Grimsgaard, S. (2010). The Acupuncture on Hot Flashes Among Menopausal Women study: Observational follow-up results at 6 and 12 months. *Menopause, 17*(2), 262-268.

Butt, D. A., Lock, M., Lewis, J. E., Ross, S., & Moineddin, R. (2008). Gabapentin for the treatment of menopausal hot flashes: A randomized controlled trial. *Menopause, 15*(2), 310-318.

Carroll, D. G., & Kelley, K. W. (2009). Use of antidepressants for management of hot flashes. *Pharmacotherapy, 29*(11), 1357-1374.

D'Anna, R., Cannata, M. L., Atteritano, M., Cancellieri, F., Corrado, F., Baviera, G., et al. (2007). Effects of the phytoestrogen genistein on hot flushes, endometrium, and vaginal epithelium in postmenopausal women: A 1-year randomized, double-blind, placebo-controlled study. *Menopause, 14*(4), 648-655.

Dog, L. (2005). Menopause: A review of botanical dietary supplements. *The American Journal of Medicine, 118*(12), 98-108.

Ferrari, A. (2009). Soy extract phytoestrogens with high dose of isoflavones for menopausal symptoms. *Journal of Obstetrics and Gynaecology Research, 35*(6), 1083-1090.

Genazzani, A. R., & Pluchino, N. (2009). Menopausal hot flashes: Still an undiscovered territory. *Menopause, 16*(5), 851-853.

Grady, D. (2006). Management of menopausal symptoms. *The New England Journal of Medicine, 355*(22), 2338-2347.

Guttuso, T., Jr., Kurlan, R., McDermott, M. P., & Kieburtz, K. (2003). Gabapentin's effects on hot flashes in postmenopausal women:

A randomized controlled trial. *Obstetrics & Gynecology, 101*(2), 337–345.

Kim, K. H. O., Kang, K. W., Kim, D. I. O., Kim, H. J. O., Yoon, H. M. O., Lee, J. M. O., et al. (2010). Effects of acupuncture on hot flashes in perimenopausal and postmenopausal women—A multi-center randomized clinical trial. *Menopause, 17*(2), 269–280.

Kronenberg, F., & Fugh-Berman, A. (2002). Complementary and alternative medicine for menopausal symptoms: A review of randomized, controlled trials. *Annals of Internal Medicine, 137*(10), 805–813.

McKinlay, S. M., Brambilla, D. J., & Posner, J. G. (2008). "Reprint of" the normal menopause transition. *Maturitas, 61*(1-2), 4–16.

Mello, N. K. (2008). Commentary on black cohosh for the treatment of menopausal symptoms. *Menopause: The Journal of the North American Menopause Society, 15*(5), 819–820.

Messina, M. J., & Wood, C. E. (2008). Soy isoflavones, estrogen therapy, and breast cancer risk: Analysis and commentary. *Nutrition Journal, 7*(1), 17–28.

Messina, M., & Wu, A. H. (2009). Perspectives on the soy-breast cancer relation. *American Journal of Clinical Nutrition, 89*(5), 1673S.

Mohyi, D., Tabassi, K., & Simon, J. (1997). Differential diagnosis of hot flashes. *Maturitas, 27*(3), 203–214.

Nelson, H. D., Vesco, K. K., Haney, E., Fu, R., Nedrow, A., Miller, J., et al. (2006). Nonhormonal therapies for menopausal hot flashes: Systematic review and meta-analysis. *JAMA: The Journal of the American Medical Association, 295*(17), 2057–2071.

Philp, H. A. (2003). Hot flashes: A review of the literature on alternative and complementary treatment approaches. *Alternative Medicine Review, 8*(3), 284–302.

Seritan, A. L., Iosif, A., Park, J. H., Deatherage Hand, D. B. S. N., Sweet, R. L., & Gold, E. B. (2010). Self-reported anxiety, depressive, and vasomotor symptoms: A study of perimenopausal women presenting to a specialized midlife assessment center. *Menopause, 17*(2), 410–415.

Shen, W., & Stearns, V. (2009). Treatment strategies for hot flushes. *Expert Opinion on Pharmacotherapy, 10*(7), 1133-1144.

Statements, A. (2009). Night sweats in postmenopausal women linked to reduced 20-year mortality rate CME/CE. *Menopause, 16*, 888-891.

Stearns, V. (2006). Serotonergic agents as an alternative to hormonal therapy for the treatment of menopausal vasomotor symptoms. *Treatments in Endocrinology, 5*(2), 83-87.

Tan Garcia, J., Gonzaga, F., Tan, D., Yaa Ng, T., Ling Oei, P. M. R. C. O. G., & Chan, C. W. B. M. R. C. O. G. (2010). Use of a multibotanical (nutrafem) for the relief of menopausal vasomotor symptoms: A double-blind, placebo-controlled study. *Menopause, 17*(2), 303-308.

Thurston, R. C., Kuller, L. H. D. H., Edmundowicz, D., & Matthews, K. A. (2010). History of hot flashes and aortic calcification among postmenopausal women. *Menopause, 17*(2), 256-261.

Vincent, A., & Fitzpatrick, L. A. (2000). Soy isoflavones: Are they useful in menopause? *Mayo Clinic Proceedings, 75*(11), 1174-1184.

Chapter 4

Ancoli-Israel, S., Kripke, D. F., Klauber, M. R., Mason, W. J., Fell, R., & Kaplan, O. (1991). Sleep-disordered breathing in community-dwelling elderly. *Sleep, 14*(6), 486-495.

Bixler, E. O., Papaliaga, M. N., Vgontzas, A. N., Lin, H. M. O., Pejovic, S., Karataraki, M., et al. (2009). Women sleep objectively better than men and the sleep of young women is more resilient to external stressors: Effects of age and menopause. *Journal of Sleep Research, 18*(2), 221-228.

Buscemi, N., Vandermeer, B., Friesen, C., Bialy, L., Tubman, M., Ospina, M., et al. (2007). The efficacy and safety of drug treatments for chronic insomnia in adults: A meta-analysis of RCTs. *Journal of General Internal Medicine, 22*(9), 1335-1350.

Dancey, D. R., Hanly, P. J., Soong, C., Lee, B., & Hoffstein, V. (2001). Impact of menopause on the prevalence and severity of sleep apnea. *Chest, 120*(1), 151–155.

Earley, C. J. (2003). Restless legs syndrome. *The New England Journal of Medicine, 348*(21), 2103–2109.

Freedman, R. R., & Roehrs, T. A. (2007). Sleep disturbance in menopause. *Menopause, 14*(5), 826–829.

Kamel, N. S., & Gammack, J. K. (2006). Insomnia in the elderly: Cause, approach, and treatment. *The American Journal of Medicine, 119*(6), 463–469.

Lauderdale, D. S., Knutson, K. L., Yan, L. L., Liu, K., & Rathouz, P. J. (2008). Self-reported and measured sleep duration: How similar are they? *Epidemiology, 19*(6), 838–845.

LeBlanc, M., Beaulieu-Bonneau, S., Mérette, C., Savard, J., Ivers, H., & Morin, C. M. (2007). Psychological and health-related quality of life factors associated with insomnia in a population-based sample. *Journal of Psychosomatic Research, 63*(2), 157–166.

Mendelson, W. B., Roth, T., Cassella, J., Roehrs, T., Walsh, J. K., Woods, J. H., et al. (2004). The treatment of chronic insomnia: Drug indications, chronic use and abuse liability. *Sleep Medicine Reviews, 8*(1), 7–17.

Morgenthaler, T., Kramer, M., Alessi, C., Friedman, L., Boehlecke, B., Brown, T., et al. (2006). Practice parameters for the psychological and behavioral treatment of insomnia: An update. *Sleep, 29*(11), 1415–1419.

Morin, C. M., Bootzin, R. R., Buysse, D. J., Edinger, J. D., Espie, C. A., & Lichstein, K. L. (2006). Psychological and behavioral treatment of insomnia: Update of the recent evidence (1998–2004). *Sleep, 29*(11), 1398–1414.

Morin, C. M., Vallieres, A., Guay, B., Ivers, H., Savard, J., Merette, C., et al. (2009). Cognitive behavioral therapy, singly and combined with medication, for persistent insomnia: A randomized controlled trial. *JAMA: The Journal of the American Medical Association, 301*(19), 2005–2015.

Neubauer, D. N. (2009). New directions in the pharmacologic treatment of sleep disorders. *Primary Psychiatry, 16*(2), 52–58.

Nowakowski, S., Meliska, C. J., Fernando Martinez, L., & Parry, B. L. (2009). Sleep and menopause. *Current Neurology and Neuroscience Reports, 9*(2), 165-172.

Ondo, W. G. (2009). Restless legs syndrome. *Neurologic Clinics, 27*(3), 779-799.

Parry, B. L. (2007). Sleep disturbances at menopause are related to sleep disorders and anxiety symptoms. *Menopause, 14*(5), 812-814.

Reed, S. D., Newton, K. M., LaCroix, A. Z., Grothaus, L. C., & Ehrlich, K. (2007). Night sweats, sleep disturbance, and depression associated with diminished libido in late menopausal transition and early postmenopause: Baseline data from the Herbal Alternatives for Menopause Trial (HALT). *American Journal of Obstetrics and Gynecology, 196*(6), 593-593.

Sivertsen, B., Omvik, S., Pallesen, S., Bjorvatn, B., Havik, O. E., Kvale, G., et al. (2006). Cognitive behavioral therapy vs zopiclone for treatment of chronic primary insomnia in older adults: A randomized controlled trial. *JAMA: The Journal of the American Medical Association, 295*(24), 2851-2858.

Stepanski, E. J., & Wyatt, J. K. (2003). Use of sleep hygiene in the treatment of insomnia. *Sleep Medicine Reviews, 7*(3), 215-225.

Teran-Santos, J., Jimenez-Gomez, A., & Cordero-Guevara, J. (1999). The association between sleep apnea and the risk of traffic accidents. *The New England Journal of Medicine, 340*(11), 847-851.

Verster, J. C., Veldhuijzen, D. S., & Volkerts, E. R. (2004). Residual effects of sleep medication on driving ability. *Sleep Medicine Reviews, 8*(4), 309-325.

Wade, A. G., Ford, I., Crawford, G., McMahon, A. D., Nir, T., Laudon, M., et al. (2007). Efficacy of prolonged release melatonin in insomnia patients aged 55-80 years: Quality of sleep and next-day alertness outcomes. *Current Medical Research and Opinion, 23*(10), 2597-2605.

Young, T., Finn, L., Austin, D., & Peterson, A. (2003). Menopausal status and sleep-disordered breathing in the Wisconsin Sleep Cohort Study. *American Journal of Respiratory and Critical Care Medicine, 167*(9), 1181-1185.

Young, T., Peppard, P. E., & Gottlieb, D. J. (2002). Epidemiology of obstructive sleep apnea: A population health perspective. *American Journal of Respiratory and Critical Care Medicine, 165*(9), 1217-1239.

Chapter 5

Addis, I. B., Van Den Eeden, S. K., Wassel-Fyr, C. L., Vittinghoff, E., Brown, J. S., & Thom, D. H. (2006). Sexual activity and function in middle-aged and older women. *Obstetrics and Gynecology, 107*(4), 755-764.

Archer, D. F. (2009). Efficacy and tolerability of local estrogen therapy for urogenital atrophy. *Menopause, 17*(1), 194-203.

Avis, N. E., Brockwell, S., Randolph, J. F., Jr., Shen, S., Cain, V. S., Ory, M., et al. (2009). Longitudinal changes in sexual functioning as women transition through menopause: Results from the study of women's health across the nation. *Menopause, 16*(3), 442-452.

Bachmann, G. A., & Leiblum, S. R. (2004). The impact of hormones on menopausal sexuality: A literature review. *Menopause, 11*(1), 120-130.

Bachmann, G., Lobo, R. A., Gut, R., Nachtigall, L., & Notelovitz, M. (2008). Efficacy of low-dose estradiol vaginal tablets in the treatment of atrophic vaginitis: A randomized controlled trial. *Obstetrics & Gynecology, 111*(1), 67-76.

Berman, J. R., Berman, L. A., Werbin, T. J., & Goldstein, I. (1999). Female sexual dysfunction: Anatomy, physiology, evaluation and treatment options. *Current Opinion in Urology, 9*(6), 563-568.

Blümel, J. E., Del Pino, M., Aprikian, D., Vallejo, S., Sarrá, S., & Castelo-Branco, C. (2008). Effect of androgens combined with hormone therapy on quality of life in post-menopausal women with sexual dysfunction. *Gynecological Endocrinology, 24*(12), 691-695.

Caillouette, J. C., & Sharp, C. F. (1997). Vaginal pH as a marker for bacterial pathogens and menopausal status. *American Journal of Obstetrics and Gynecology, 176*(6), 1270-1277.

Castelo-Branco, C., Cancelo, M. J., Villero, J., Nohales, F., & Juliá, M. D. (2005). Management of post-menopausal vaginal atrophy and atrophic vaginitis. *Maturitas, 52*, 46-52.

Cleary-Goldman, J., Malone, F. D., Vidaver, J., Ball, R. H., Nyberg, D. A., Comstock, C. H., et al. (2005). Impact of maternal age on obstetric outcome. *Obstetrics & Gynecology, 105*(5, Pt. 1), 983-990.

Davis, S. R., Davison, S. L., Donath, S., & Bell, R. J. (2005). Circulating androgen levels and self-reported sexual function in women. *JAMA: The Journal of the American Medical Association, 294*(1), 91-96.

Davison, S. L., Bell, R., Donath, S., Montalto, J. G., & Davis, S. R. (2005). Androgen levels in adult females: Changes with age, menopause, and oophorectomy. *Journal of Clinical Endocrinology & Metabolism, 90*(7), 3847-3853.

Freedman, M. (2008). Vaginal pH, estrogen and genital atrophy. *Menopause Management, 17*(4), 9-13.

Hayes, R., & Dennerstein, L. (2005). The impact of aging on sexual function and sexual dysfunction in women: A review of population-based studies. *The Journal of Sexual Medicine, 2*(3), 317-330.

Heiman, J. R. (2008). Treating low sexual desire—New findings for testosterone in women. *New England Journal of Medicine, 359*(19), 2047-2049.

Huang, A. J., Moore, E. E., Boyko, E. J., Scholes, D., Lin, F., Vittinghoff, E., et al. (2010). Vaginal symptoms in postmenopausal women: Self-reported severity, natural history, and risk factors. *Menopause, 17*(1), 121-126.

Katz, A. (2007). When sex hurts: Menopause-related dyspareunia. *The American Journal of Nursing, 107*(7), 34-36, 39.

Li, C., Samsioe, G., Borgfeldt, C., Lidfeldt, J., Agardh, C. D., & Nerbrand, C. (2003). Menopause-related symptoms: What are the background factors? A prospective population-based cohort study of Swedish women (the Women's Health in Lund Area study). *American Journal of Obstetrics and Gynecology, 189*(6), 1646-1653.

Lindau, S. T., Schumm, L. P., Laumann, E. O., Levinson, W., O'Muircheartaigh, C. A., & Waite, L. J. (2007). A study of sexuality and health among older adults in the United States. *The New England Journal of Medicine, 357*(8), 762-774.

NAMS. (2007). The role of vaginal estrogen for treatment of vaginal atrophy in postmenopausal women: 2007 position statement of the North American Menopause Society. *Menopause, 14*(3), 357-369.

Panjari, M., Bell, R. J., Jane, F., Wolfe, R., Adams, J., Morrow, C., et al. (2009). A randomized trial of oral DHEA treatment for sexual function, well-being, and menopausal symptoms in postmenopausal women with low libido. *The Journal of Sexual Medicine, 6*(9), 2579-2590.

Panjari, M., & Davis, S. R. (2007). DHEA therapy for women: Effect on sexual function and wellbeing. *Human Reproduction Update, 13*, 239-248.

Panzer, C., & Guay, A. (2009). Testosterone replacement therapy in naturally and surgically menopausal women. *Journal of Sexual Medicine, 6*, 8-18.

Patel, S. M., Ratcliffe, S. J., Reilly, M. P., Weinstein, R., Bhasin, S., Blackman, M. R., et al. (2009). Higher serum testosterone concentration in older women is associated with insulin resistance, metabolic syndrome, and cardiovascular disease. *Journal of Clinical Endocrinology & Metabolism, 94*(12), 4776-4784.

Phillips, E. H., Ryan, S., Ferrari, R., & Green, C. (2003). Estratest® and Estratest® HS (esterified estrogens and methyltestosterone) therapy: A summary of safety surveillance data, January 1989 to August 2002. *Clinical Therapeutics, 25*(12), 3027-3043.

Riphagen, F. E., Fortney, J. A., & Koelb, S. (2008). Contraception in women over forty. *Journal of Biosocial Science, 20*(2), 127-142.

Schover, L. R. (2008). Androgen therapy for loss of desire in women: Is the benefit worth the breast cancer risk? *Fertility and Sterility, 90*(1), 129-140.

Seibert, C., Barbouche, E., Fagan, J., Myint, E., Wetterneck, T., & Wittemyer, M. (2003). Prescribing oral contraceptives for women older than 35 years of age. *Annals of Internal Medicine, 138,* 54-64.

Somboonporn, W. (2007). Emerging role of testosterone in menopause. *Women's Health, 3*(6), 663-665.

Tarcan, T., Park, K., Goldstein, I., Maio, G., Fassina, A., Krane, R. J., et al. (1999). Histomorphometric analysis of age-related structural changes in human clitoral cavernosal tissue. *The Journal of Urology, 161*(3), 940-944.

Williams, J. K. (2002). Contraceptive needs of the perimenopausal woman. *Obstetrics and Gynecology Clinics of North America, 29*(3), 575-588.

Chapter 6

Bonaiuti, D., Shea, B., Iovine, R., Negrini, S., Robinson, V., Kemper, H., et al. (2002). Exercise for preventing and treating osteoporosis in postmenopausal women. *Cochrane Database of Systematic Reviews, 3*(3). Retrieved August 2, 2010, from http://ezproxy.library.nyu.edu:2538/cochrane/clsysrev/articles/CD000333/pdf_fs.html

Chesnut III, C. H., Silverman, S., Andriano, K., Genant, H., Gimona, A., Harris, S., et al. (2000). A randomized trial of nasal spray salmon calcitonin in postmenopausal women with established osteoporosis: The prevent recurrence of osteoporotic fractures study. *The American Journal of Medicine, 109*(4), 267-276.

Compston, J. E. (2010). Bisphosphonates and atypical femoral fractures: A time for reflection. *Maturitas, 65*(1), 3-4.

Francis, R. M., Aspray, T. J., Hide, G., Sutcliffe, A. M., & Wilkinson, P. (2008). Back pain in osteoporotic vertebral fractures. *Osteoporosis International, 19*(7), 895-903.

Gallagher, J. C. (2007). Effect of early menopause on bone mineral density and fractures. *Menopause, 14*(3), 567-571.

Gass, M., & Dawson-Hughes, B. (2006). Preventing osteoporosis-related fractures: An overview. *The American Journal of Medicine, 119*(4, Suppl. 1), 3-11.

Hathcock, J. N., Shao, A., Vieth, R., & Heaney, R. (2007). Risk assessment for vitamin D. *American Journal of Clinical Nutrition, 85*(1), 6.

Holick, M. F. (2007). Vitamin D deficiency. *The New England Journal of Medicine, 357*(3), 266-281.

Khosla, S. (2009). Increasing options for the treatment of osteoporosis. *The New England Journal of Medicine, 361*(8), 818-820.

Khosla, S., Burr, D., Cauley, J., Dempster, D. W., Ebeling, P. R., Felsenberg, D., et al. (2007). Bisphosphonate-associated osteonecrosis of the jaw: Report of a task force of the American society for bone and mineral research. *Journal of Bone and Mineral Research, 22*, 1479-1491.

Knopp, J. A., Diner, B. M., Blitz, M., Lyritis, G. P., & Rowe, B. H. (2005). Calcitonin for treating acute pain of osteoporotic vertebral compression fractures: A systematic review of randomized, controlled trials. *Osteoporosis International, 16*(10), 1281-1290.

Melton III, L. J., Chrischilles, E. A., Cooper, C., Lane, A. W., & Riggs, B. L. (2005). How many women have osteoporosis? *Journal of Bone and Mineral Research, 20*(5), 886-892.

NAMS. (2010). Management of osteoporosis in postmenopausal women: 2010 position statement of The North American Menopause Society. *Menopause: The Journal of The North American Menopause Society, 17*(1), 25-54.

Nguyen, T. V., Kelly, P. J., Sambrook, P. N., Gilbert, C., Pocock, N. A., & Eisman, J. A. (2009). Lifestyle factors and bone density in the elderly: Implications for osteoporosis prevention. *Journal of Bone and Mineral Research, 9*(9), 1339-1346.

Schwab, P., & Klein, R. F. (2008). Nonpharmacological approaches to improve bone health and reduce osteoporosis. *Current Opinion in Rheumatology, 20*(2), 213-217.

Shane, E. (2010). Evolving data about subtrochanteric fractures and bisphosphonates. *The New England Journal of Medicine.* Retrieved April 1, 2010, from www.nejm.org

Soroko, S. B., Barrett-Connor, E., Edelstein, S. L., & Kritz-Silverstein, D. (2009). Family history of osteoporosis and bone mineral density at the axial skeleton: The Rancho Bernardo study. *Journal of Bone and Mineral Research, 9*(6), 761-769.

Vainionpää, A., Korpelainen, R., Sievänen, H., Vihriälä, E., Leppäluoto, J., & Jämsä, T. (2007). Effect of impact exercise and its intensity on bone geometry at weight-bearing tibia and femur. *Bone, 40*(3), 604-611.

Vieth, R., Bischoff-Ferrari, H., Boucher, B. J., Dawson-Hughes, B., Garland, C. F., Heaney, R. P., et al. (2007). The urgent need to recommend an intake of vitamin D that is effective. *American Journal of Clinical Nutrition, 85*(3), 649-650.

Wang, T. J., Pencina, M. J., Booth, S. L., Jacques, P. F., Ingelsson, E., Lanier, K., et al. (2008). Vitamin D deficiency and risk of cardiovascular disease. *Circulation, 117*(4), 503-511.

Zittermann, A. (2007). Vitamin D in preventive medicine: Are we ignoring the evidence? *British Journal of Nutrition, 89*(5), 552-572.

Chapter 7

AACE Menopause Guidelines Revision Task Force. (2006). American Association of Clinical Endocrinologists medical guidelines for clinical practice for the diagnosis and treatment of menopause. *Endocrine Practice, 12*(3), 315-337.

Archer, D. F. (2005). Progestogens: Effects on clinical and biochemical parameters in postmenopausal women. *Menopause, 12*(5), 484-487.

Banks, E. (2002). From dogs' testicles to mares' urine: The origins and contemporary use of hormonal therapy for the menopause. *Feminist Review, 72*, 2-25.

FDA. (2009). *Estrogen and estrogen with progestin therapies for postmenopausal women.* Retrieved February 7, 2010, from http://www.fda.gov/Drugs/DrugSafety/InformationbyDrugClass/ucm135318.htm

Gruber, C. J., Tschugguel, W., Schneeberger, C., & Huber, J. C. (2002). Production and actions of estrogens. *The New England Journal of Medicine, 346*(5), 340-352.

Heiss, G., Wallace, R., Anderson, G. L., Aragaki, A., Beresford, S. A. A., Brzyski, R., et al. (2008). Health risks and benefits 3 years after stopping randomized treatment with estrogen and progestin. *JAMA: The Journal of the American Medical Association, 299*(9), 1036-1045.

McCrea, F. B. (1983). The politics of menopause: The "discovery" of a deficiency disease. *Social Problems, 31*(1), 111-123.

Menon, U., Burnell, M., Sharma, A., Gentry-Maharaj, A., Fraser, L., Ryan, A., Parmar, M., Hunter, M., & Jacobs, I. (2007). Decline in use of hormone therapy among postmenopausal women in the United Kingdom. *Menopause, 14*(3), 462-467.

NAMS. (2010). Estrogen and progestogen use in postmenopausal women: 2010 position statement of The North American Menopause Society. *Menopause: The Journal of The North American Menopause Society, 17*(2), 242-255.

Neugarten, B. L., Wood, V., Kraines, R. J., & Loomis, B. (1964). Women's attitudes toward the menopause. *Obstetrical & Gynecological Survey, 19*(1), 149-151.

Panjari, M., & Davis, S. R. (2007). DHEA therapy for women: Effect on sexual function and wellbeing. *Human Reproduction Update, 13*(3), 239-248.

Pearl, M. J., & Plotz, E. J. (1964). Management of the climacteric patient. *Clinical Obstetrics and Gynecology, 7*(2), 476-488.

Ravdin, P. M., Cronin, K. A., Howlader, N., Berg, C. D., Chlebowski, R. T., Feuer, E. J., Edwards, B. K., & Berry, D. A. (2007). The decrease in breast-cancer incidence in 2003 in the United States. *The New England Journal of Medicine, 356*(16), 1670-1674.

Rossouw, J. E., Anderson, G. L., Prentice, R. L., LaCroix, A. Z., Kooperberg, C., Stefanick, M. L., Jackson, R. D., Beresford, S. A., Howard, B. V., & Johnson, K. C. (2002). Risks and benefits of estrogen plus progestin in healthy postmenopausal women: Principal results from the Women's Health Initiative randomized controlled trial. *JAMA: The Journal of the American Medical Association, 288*(3), 321-333.

Ruggiero, R. J., & Likis, F. E. (2002). Estrogen: Physiology, pharmacology, and formulations for replacement therapy. *Journal of Midwifery & Women's Health, 47*(3), 130-138.

Smith, D. C., Prentice, R., Thompson, D. J., & Herrmann, W. L. (1975). Association of exogenous estrogen and endometrial cancer. *The New England Journal of Medicine, 293*(23), 1164-1167.

Wilson, R. A. (1964). The obsolete menopause. *Delaware Medical Journal, 36*, 20-21.

Wilson, R. A., Brevetti, R. E., & Wilson, T. A. (1963). Specific procedures for the elimination of the menopause. *Western Journal of Surgery, Obstetrics, and Gynecology, 71*(1), 110-121.

Wilson, R. A., & Wilson, T. A. (1963). The fate of the nontreated postmenopausal woman: A plea for the maintenance of adequate estrogen from puberty to the grave. *Journal of the American Geriatrics Society, 11*, 347-362.

Women's Health Initiative Steering Committee. (2004). Effects of conjugated equine estrogen in postmenopausal women with hysterectomy. *JAMA: The Journal of the American Medical Association, 291*(14), 1701-1712.

Ziel, H. K., & Finkle, W. D. (1975). Increased risk of endometrial cancer among users of conjugated estrogens. *The New England Journal of Medicine, 293*, 1167-1170.

Chapter 8

AACE Menopause Guidelines Revision Task Force. (2006). American Association of Clinical Endocrinologists medical guidelines for clinical practice for the diagnosis and treatment of menopause. *Endocrine Practice, 12*(3), 315-337.

AHRQ. (2008). *Menopause and hormone therapy (HT): Collaborative decision-making and management.* Retrieved March 5, 2010 from http://www.guideline.gov/summary/summary.aspx?view_id=1&doc_id=13312

Altman, A. M. (2007). Bioidentical hormones: What's fact and what's fable? *Sexuality, Reproduction & Menopause, 5*(1), 14.

Archer, D. F. (2005). Progestogens: Effects on clinical and bio-chemical parameters in postmenopausal women. *Menopause, 12*(5), 484-487.

Birkhäuser, M. H., Birkhäuser, M. H., Panay, N., Archer, D. F., Barlow, D., Burger, H., Gambacciani, M., Goldstein, S., Pinkerton, J. A., & Sturdee, D. W. (2008). Updated practical rec-ommendations for hormone replacement therapy in the peri- and postmenopause. *Climacteric, 11*(2), 108-123.

Bosarge, P. M., & Freeman, S. (2009). Bioidentical hormones, com-pounding, and evidence-based medicine: What women's health practitioners need to know. *Journal for Nurse Practitioners, 5*(6), 421-427.

Chervenak, J. (2009). Bioidentical hormones for maturing women. *Maturitas, 64*(2), 86-89.

Cirigliano, M. (2007). Bioidentical hormone therapy: A review of the evidence. *Journal of Women's Health, 16*(5), 600-631.

Davison, S. (2009). Salivary testing opens a Pandora's box of issues surrounding accurate measurement of testosterone in women. *Menopause, 16*(4), 630-631.

Grady, D. (2006). Management of menopausal symptoms. *The New England Journal of Medicine, 355*(22), 2338-2347.

Gruber, C. J., Tschugguel, W., Schneeberger, C., & Huber, J. C. (2002). Production and actions of estrogens. *The New England Journal of Medicine, 346*(5), 340-352.

Haskell, S. G., Bean-Mayberry, B., & Gordon, K. (2009). Discontinuing postmenopausal hormone therapy: An obser-vational study of tapering versus quitting cold turkey: Is there a difference in recurrence of menopausal symptoms? *Menopause, 16*(3), 494-499.

Heiss, G., Wallace, R., Anderson, G. L., Aragaki, A., Beresford, S. A. A., Brzyski, R., Chlebowski, R. T., Gass, M., LaCroix, A., & Manson, J. A. E. (2008). Health risks and benefits 3 years after stop-ping randomized treatment with estrogen and progestin. *JAMA: The Journal of the American Medical Association, 299*(9), 1036-1045.

Jaakkola, S., Lyytinen, H., Pukkala, E., & Ylikorkala, O. (2009). Endometrial cancer in postmenopausal women using estradiol-progestin therapy. *Obstetrics & Gynecology, 114*(6), 1197-1204.

Practice Committee of the American Society for Reproductive Medicine. (2006). Estrogen and progestogen therapy in post-menopausal women. *Fertility and Sterility, 86*, 4.

Rossouw, J. E., Anderson, G. L., Prentice, R. L., LaCroix, A. Z., Kooperberg, C., Stefanick, M. L., et al. (2002). Risks and benefits of estrogen plus progestin in healthy postmenopausal women: Principal results from the women's health initiative randomized controlled trial. *JAMA: The Journal of the American Medical Association, 288*(3), 321-333.

Ruggiero, R. J., & Likis, F. E. (2002). Estrogen: Physiology, pharmacology, and formulations for replacement therapy. *Journal of Midwifery & Women's Health, 47*(3), 130-138.

Women's Health Initiative Steering Committee. (2004). Effects of conjugated equine estrogen in postmenopausal women with hysterectomy. *JAMA: The Journal of the American Medical Association, 291*, 1701-1712.

Chapter 9

Aston, J. L., Lodolce, A. E., & Shapiro, N. L. (2006). Interaction between warfarin and cranberry juice. *Pharmacotherapy, 26*(9), 1314-1319.

Bibbins-Domingo, K., Chertow, G. M., Coxson, P. G., Moran, A., Lightwood, J. M., Pletcher, M. J., et al. (2010). Projected effect of dietary salt reductions on future cardiovascular disease. *New England Journal of Medicine 362*, 590-599.

Cleeman, J. I. (2001). Executive summary of the third report of the National Cholesterol Education Program (NCEP) Expert Panel on Detection, Evaluation, and Treatment of High Blood Cholesterol in Adults (Adult Treatment Panel III). *Journal of the American Medical Association, 285*(19), 2486-2497.

Djousse, L., & Lee, I. (2009). Alcohol consumption and risk of cardiovascular disease and death in women: Potential mediating mechanisms. *Circulation, 120*(3), 237-244.

Epstein, E., & Valentin, L. (2004). Managing women with post-menopausal bleeding. *Best Practice & Research Clinical Obstetrics & Gynaecology, 18*(1), 125-143.

Fox, K. R. (2007). The influence of physical activity on mental well-being. *Public Health Nutrition, 2*(3a), 411-418.

Freeman, E. W., Sammel, M. D., Lin, H., Gracia, C. R., & Kapoor, S. (2008). Symptoms in the menopausal transition: Hormone and behavioral correlates. *Obstetrics & Gynecology, 111*(1), 127-136.

Geller, S. E., & Studee, L. (2007). Botanical and dietary supplements for mood and anxiety in menopausal women. *Menopause, 14*(3), 541-549.

Greendale, G. A., Huang, M. H., Wight, R. G., Seeman, T., Luetters, C., Avis, N. E., et al. (2009). Effects of the menopause transition and hormone use on cognitive performance in midlife women. *Neurology, 72*(21), 1850-1857.

Grushka, M., Epstein, J. B., & Gorsky, M. (2002). Burning mouth syndrome. *American Family Physician, 65*(4), 615-621.

Hsu, C. Y., Chen, C. P., & Wang, K. L. (2008). Assessment of post-menopausal bleeding. *International Journal of Gerontology, 2*(2), 55-59.

Innes, K. E., Selfe, T. K., & Taylor, A. G. (2008). Menopause, the metabolic syndrome, and mind–body therapies. *Menopause, 15*(5), 1005-1013.

Janssen, I., Powell, L. H., Crawford, S., Lasley, B., & Sutton-Tyrrell, K. (2008). Menopause and the metabolic syndrome: The study of women's health across the nation. *Archives of Internal Medicine, 168*(14), 1568-1575.

Jepson, R. G., Mihaljevic, L., & Craig, J. (2004). Cranberries for preventing urinary tract infections. *Cochrane Database of Systematic Reviews, 2*, 1-19.

Kontiokari, T., Sundqvist, K., Nuutinen, M., Pokka, T., Koskela, M., & Uhari, M. (2001). Randomised trial of cranberry-lingonberry juice and *Lactobacillus* GG drink for the prevention of urinary tract infections in women. *British Medical Journal, 322*(7302), 1571.

MacGregor, E. A. (2009). Estrogen replacement and migraine. *Maturitas, 63*(1), 51–55.

Maki, P. M. (2008). Menopause and anxiety: Immediate and long-term effects. *Menopause, 15*(6), 1033–1035.

Meisel, P., Reifenberger, J., Haase, R., Nauck, M., Bandt, C., & Kocher, T. (2008). Women are periodontally healthier than men, but why don't they have more teeth than men? *Menopause, 15*(2), 270–275.

Nelson, H. D., Tyne, K., Naik, A., Bougatsos, C., Chan, B. K., & Humphrey, L. (2009). Screening for breast cancer: An update for the US preventive services task force. *Annals of Internal Medicine, 151*(10), 727–737.

Partridge, E., Kreimer, A. R., Greenlee, R. T., Williams, C., Xu, J. L., Church, T. R., et al. (2009). Results from four rounds of ovarian cancer screening in a randomized trial. *Obstetrical & Gynecological Survey, 64*(9), 593–595.

Penedo, F. J., & Dahn, J. R. (2005). Exercise and well-being: A review of mental and physical health benefits associated with physical activity. *Current Opinion in Psychiatry, 18*(2), 189–193.

Pines, A., & Berry, E. M. (2007). Exercise in the menopause—An update. *Climacteric, 10*, 42–46.

Raz, R., Chazan, B., & Dan, M. (2004). Cranberry juice and urinary tract infection. *Clinical Infectious Diseases, 38*, 1413–1419.

Rosano, G. M. C., Vitale, C., Marazzi, G., & Volterrani, M. (2007). Menopause and cardiovascular disease: The evidence. *Climacteric, 10*, 19–24.

Schenck-Gustafsson, K. (2009). Risk factors for cardiovascular disease in women. *Maturitas, 63*(3), 186–190.

Smith, R. A., Cokkinides, V., Brooks, D., Saslow, D., & Brawley, O. W. (2010). Cancer screening in the United States, 2010: A review of current American Cancer Society guidelines and issues in cancer screening. *CA: A Cancer Journal for Clinicians, 60*(2), 99–199.

Szoeke, C. E., Cicuttini, F. M., Guthrie, J. R., & Dennerstein, L. (2008). The relationship of reports of aches and joint pains to the menopausal transition: A longitudinal study. *Climacteric, 11*(1), 55–62.

Szoeke, C. E. I., Cicuttini, F., Guthrie, J., & Dennerstein, L. (2005). Self-reported arthritis and the menopause. *Climacteric, 8*(1), 49–55.

Tangen, T., & Mykletun, A. (2008). Depression and anxiety through the climacteric period: An epidemiological study (HUNT-II). *Journal of Psychosomatic Obstetrics & Gynecology, 29*(2), 125–131.

Tankó, L. B., Karsdal, M. A., & Christiansen, C. (2005). The clinical potential of estrogen for the prevention of osteoarthritis: What is known and what needs to be done? *Womens Health, 1*(1), 125–132.

Turner, M. D., & Ship, J. A. (2007). Dry mouth and its effects on the oral health of elderly people. *The Journal of the American Dental Association, 138*(1), 15S.

Waetjen, L. E., Ye, J., Feng, W. Y., Johnson, W. O., Greendale, G. A., Sampselle, C. M., et al. (2009). Association between menopausal transition stages and developing urinary incontinence. *Obstetrics & Gynecology, 114*(5), 989–998.

Weber, M., & Mapstone, M. (2009). Memory complaints and memory performance in the menopausal transition. *Menopause, 16*(4), 694–700.

Wildman, R. P., Colvin, A. B., Powell, L. H., Matthews, K. A., Everson-Rose, S. A., Hollenberg, S., et al. (2008). Associations of endogenous sex hormones with the vasculature in menopausal women: The Study of Women's Health Across the Nation (SWAN). *Menopause, 15*(3), 414–421.

Chapter 10

Bopp, M. J., Houston, D. K., Lenchik, L., Easter, L., Kritchevsky, S. B., & Nicklas, B. J. (2008). Lean mass loss is associated with low protein intake during dietary-induced weight loss in postmenopausal women. *Journal of the American Dietetic Association, 108*(7), 1216–1220.

Brincat, M. P., Baron, Y. M., & Galea, R. (2005). Estrogens and the skin. *Climacteric, 8*(2), 110–123.

Cheng, M. H., Wang, S. J., Yang, F. Y., Wang, P. H., & Fuh, J. L. (2009). Menopause and physical performance—A community-based cross-sectional study. *Menopause, 16*(5), 892-896.

Dansinger, M. L., Gleason, J. A., Griffith, J. L., Selker, H. P., & Schaefer, E. J. (2005). Comparison of the Atkins, Ornish, Weight Watchers, and Zone diets for weight loss and heart disease risk reduction a randomized trial. *JAMA: The Journal of the American Medical Association, 293*(1), 43-53.

Haskell, W. L., Lee, I. M., Pate, R. R., Powell, K. E., Blair, S. N., Franklin, B. A., et al. (2007). Physical activity and public health: Updated recommendation for adults from the American College of Sports Medicine and the American Heart Association. *Circulation, 116*(9), 1081-1093.

Kemmler, W., Lauber, D., Weineck, J., Hensen, J., Kalender, W., & Engelke, K. (2004). Benefits of 2 years of intense exercise on bone density, physical fitness, and blood lipids in early postmenopausal osteopenic women: Results of the Erlangen Fitness Osteoporosis Prevention Study (EFOPS). *Archives of Internal Medicine, 164*(10), 1084-1091.

Lee, I. (2010). Physical activity and weight gain prevention. *JAMA: The Journal of the American Medical Association, 303*(12), 1173-1179.

Pines, A., & Berry, E. M. (2007). Exercise in the menopause—An update. *Climacteric, 10*, 42-46.

Slaven, L., & Lee, C. (1994). Psychological effects of exercise among adult women: The impact of menopausal status. *Psychology & Health, 9*(4), 297-303.

Tsai, A. G., & Wadden, T. A. (2005). Systematic review: An evaluation of major commercial weight loss programs in the United States. *Annals of Internal Medicine, 142*(1), 56-66.

Youn, C. S., Kwon, O. S., Won, C. H., Hwang, E. J., Park, B. J., Eun, H. C., et al. (2003). Effect of pregnancy and menopause on facial wrinkling in women. *Acta Dermato-Venereologica, 83*(6), 419-424.

Index